A Handbook of Men's Health

For Churchill Livingstone:

Associate Editor: Main McCubbin
Development Editor: Claire Wilson
Project Manager: Andrew Palfreyman
Design: Stewart Larking

A Handbook of Men's Health

Tom Laws

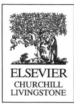

ELSEVIER
CHURCHILL
LIVINGSTONE

EDINBURGH LONDON NEW YORK OXFORD PHILADELPHIA ST LOUIS SYDNEY
TORONTO 2006

CHURCHILL LIVINGSTONE
An imprint of Elsevier Limited

The right of Tom Laws to be identified as Author of this work have been asserted by him in accordance with the Copyright, Designs and Patents Act 1988

First published 2006

ISBN 0 443 073384

British Library Cataloguing in Publication Data
A catalogue record for this book is available from the British Library

Library of Congress Cataloging in Publication Data
A catalog record for this book is available from the Library of Congress

Note
Knowledge and best practice in this field are constantly changing. As new research and experience broaden our knowledge, changes in practice, treatment and drug therapy may become necessary or appropriate. Readers are advised to check the most current information provided (i) on procedures featured or (ii) by the manufacturer of each product to be administered, to verify the recommended dose or formula, the method and duration of administration, and contraindications. It is the responsibility of the practitioner, relying on their own experience and knowledge of the patient, to make diagnoses, to determine dosages and the best treatment for each individual patient, and to take all appropriate safety precautions.
   To the fullest extent of the law, neither the publisher nor the Editors assume any liability for any injury and/or damage.

The Publisher

The
Publisher's
policy is to use
paper manufactured
from sustainable forests

Contents

Preface

WHAT IS MEN'S HEALTH?

The term 'men's health' is a banner under which its proponents espouse a number of issues. Medical science and clinical medicine have used the term in relation to researching sex-specific illness and exploring issues that men hold in relation to understanding what is happening to their bodies when a disorder, illness or disease arises. In keeping with this approach Fletcher (2001, p. 68) has narrowly defined a men's health issue as: '*a disease or condition unique to men, more prevalent in men, more serious among men, for which risk factors are different for men or for which different interventions are required.*' The complexity of the term becomes evident when gender and the socialisation of males are incorporated. A broader and more socially orientated definition of 'men's health issues' reads: 'Drawing these elements together leads to a definition of a men's health issue as any issue, condition or determinant that affects the quality of life of men and/or for which different responses are required in order for men (and boys) to experience optimal social, emotional and physical health.' (New South Wales (NSW) Department of Health website)

WHY IS MEN'S HEALTH AN ISSUE?

A central theme within women's health and men's health discourse is the need for equity between the sexes. Specifically, equality of access to health services and equity in access to resources that promote health are important issues for women. However, equity is not fully achieved by simply allocating the same amount of resources to each sex. Rather, the issue of equity is best resolved through the development of an understanding of how men and women differ socially and biologically and thereby allocating resources to meet those unique needs. The unique sexual biology and diverse social experiences of men and women give rise to different health concerns. Therefore different responses are required by health providers within a health system to meet needs and optimise health of the individual and of populations (NSW Department of Health 2000).

Developing countries

The issue of gender equity in relation to developing countries is also recognised by the World Health Organization (WHO). WHO (1998) notes that health policies and programmes have, for the most part, focused on biological aspects of diagnosis, treatment and prevention. Moreover, there is a tendency to emphasise biological or sex differences to explain factors of wellbeing and illness. The WHO technical paper 'Gender and Health' (1998) explores the critical roles that social and cultural factors and power relations between men and women play in promoting and protecting health.

The theoretical basis for gendered health

The political and theoretical trajectory of men's health differs markedly to that of the women's health movement. Feminist theory identified patriarchy as a social force oppressing women as a basis for:

- women's dissatisfaction with broad-based health services available to them
- the devaluation of women's life experiences and knowledge of health, making it difficult for them to participate fully in decisions concerning treatment.

Men's health issues have not been fundamentally supported by an overarching social theory linking gender and power to health status, although it can be said that hegemony, the domination of one class over another or domination of capitalists over the working class, plays an important part in limiting men's life choices and has negative health effects (Connell 1995). An understanding of hegemony can be gained from the literature exploring the lives of men and their families in industrial and post-industrial society. (It is useful to refer to the Oxford Dictionary of Sociology (Marshall 1998) for a primary understanding of these ideologies and concepts). In contrast with women's health, proponents of men's health issues make claims of inequity based largely on epidemiological evidence indicating that men, on average, live shorter lives than women. However, the burden of morbidity weighs heavier on women because they have chronic conditions over longer periods of their lifespan. Proponents of men's health concerns also raise the issue of higher sex differentials for accident and injury rates, referring to 'risk taking' by males as only a partial explanation for this phenomenon. Connell & Huggins (1998) contend that although there is clear recognition of the biological causes of ill health among men, the challenge for policy makers is to account for the ways in which masculinity shapes men's social behaviours and health practices.

Policy development

Many Western governments have developed national policies aimed specifically at improving women's health (Doyal 1998); however, the formulation of any substantive men's health policies is still in progress (e.g. UK, Australia, New Zealand). In the UK the Men's Health Forum has taken the initiative of launching, at the 12th Annual Public Health Forum in Brighton, a broad-based programme for policy development. The 'Getting It Sorted' policy report (Men's Health Forum 2002) sets out the steps needed to bring about significant improvements in the health of this half of the population.

However, Baker (2002) from the Health Development Agency (HDA) asserts that: 'Despite increasing interest in men's health, specific health initiatives aimed at men remain rare . . . Primary health care trusts are, as yet, showing few signs of interest. Some health promotion units have launched innovative projects, but these are often short lived and not properly evaluated'.

In Australia, four of the six state governments and one territory government ran a policy process between 1995 and 2002 resulting only in written statements about men's health. In 1996 a national men's health policy was drafted. None of the statements or the draft policy have been enacted by parliament. Lumb (2003) suggests stagnation of policy has occurred because:

- the focus has been on treating the body rather than understanding social ills;
- men are letting the data speak for them with little movement beyond;
- women became feminists to advance their cause, men have no similar social movement;

- men's health activists are seeking change at a time when health budgets generally are under pressure.

Men's health programmes in many countries have been developed by specific agencies, rather than being centrally planned and based on agreed aims and measurable outcomes. This approach, combined with a lack of ongoing funding, has meant that most men's health programmes have not been sustainable.

NURSING IN A MEN'S HEALTH CONTEXT

Over the last decade there has been an increasing awareness among health professionals of 'men's health' issues. This awareness has been driven by research literature appearing in journals for nurses and allied health professionals and by media coverage of men's health problems. By far the largest volume of research centres on the study of male-specific health problems and, to lesser extent, their impact on men's quality of life and masculinity. The experiences of men with prostate cancer and testicular cancer, including their need to understand diagnostic options and consequences of treatment, feature prominently in this respect. However, as the focus of the men's health literature widens, there is likely to be a greater understanding of the way in which gender influences men's experience of illness, disability, rehabilitation, healthcare systems in general and changes in their health status across the life span. In the current state of play, health professionals who are convinced that gender has a substantial impact on the health of individuals and groups are reliant on using multiple forms of knowledge to practise in a gender-sensitive manner.

Nurses seeking to locate literature that links gender to health status and clinical outcomes should note that research in this area is formative. Trevett's (2002) comment exemplifies this point: 'gender is rarely mentioned in either qualitative or quantitative studies, even where it appears to be an obvious factor – for example, in the incidence, cause and methods of suicide. Sometimes differences are noted, but not explored'.

USING THIS BOOK

This handbook is intended to be a first point of reference for those seeking to understand the nexus between gender, health status and health practice. The book contains a comprehensive set of topics that reflect contemporary health issues for young to older men. Consequently, the majority of the content has been structured on the basis of important junctures in the male life span. For example, there are chapters focusing on young men, prime time and maturity. Nursing interventions and biomedical matters appear in the quick reference chapters towards the end of the handbook; these chapters focus on common conditions and disorders, and some common treatments, procedures and investigations.

Aside from specific illnesses, there are important chapters dealing with health promotion, reproductive issues and a specific chapter informing on sensitive health issues. The latter provides the nurse with a valuable overview of the male reproductive issues (e.g. circumcision, sex abuse, premature ejaculation, erectile dysfunction). In-depth social analysis in terms of the causes and precursors of health problems has been avoided. Instead, the focus is primarily on the nurse as a patient advocate with the intent of enabling patients to make informed decisions about their health, medical investigations and treatments.

In almost every chapter of the handbook there are reflective exercises raising issues related to nursing care and encouraging the reader to 'spend some time thinking about the following'. For example, in the chapter on ethico-legal issues nurses are asked to reflect on issues they may hold in relation to homosexuality. This form of reflection is an important aspect of professional practice because it allows readers to become aware of how their values and beliefs may covertly influence the type and quality of care they provide. Reflexivity, where nurses scrutinise their actions and reflections within the framework of their professional role (determined by statutary declarations, guidelines and standards), has been openly encouraged as a useful tool for enhancing clinical practice (Peerson & Yong 2003).

Tom Laws
Adelaide, 2005

Reference

Baker P 2002 Health Development Agency website. Comment: Men need more support. Online. Available: http://www.hda-online.org.uk/hdt/0602/comment2.html

Connell RW 1995 Masculinities. Hartnolls, Bodmin

Connell R, Huggins A 1998 Men's health; health policy is beginning to recognise issues of masculinity. Medical Journal of Australia 169 (6): 295–296

Doyal L 1998 Introduction: women and health services. In: Doyal L (ed) Women and health services. Open University Press, Milton Keynes

Fletcher R 2001 The development of men's health in Australia. In: Davidson N, Lloyd T (eds) Promoting men's health: a guide for practitioners. Baillière Tindall, Edinburgh

Lumb P 2003 Why is men's health and well-being policy not implemented in Australia? International Journal of Men's Health 2(1): 73–86

Marshall G (ed) 1998 Oxford dictionary of sociology. Oxford University Press, New York

Men's Health Forum 2002 Getting it sorted: a new policy for men's health. The Men's Health Forum, London. Online. Available: http://www.menshealthforum.org.uk/uploaded_files/gettingsorted2002.pdf

NSW Department of Health 1999 Moving forwards in men's health. State Health Publication No (HSP) 990064. Online. Available: http://www.health.nsw.gov.au/health-public-affairs/men'shealth/pdf/men's health.pdf

NSW Department of Health 2000 Gender equity in health: better health good health care. Better Health: Publications Warehouse, Gladesville, New South Wales. Online. Available: http://www.health.nsw.gov.au/health-public-affairs/bhc/bhc.html

Peerson A, Yong V 2003 Reflexivity in nursing: where is the patient? Where is the nurse? Australian Journal of Holistic Nursing 10(1): 30–45

Trevett N 2002 Mind the gender gap. Health Development Agency. (Feb/March). Online. Available: http://www.hda-online.org.uk/hdt/0102/evidence.html

World Health Organisation 1998 Gender and health: Introduction. Technical paper WHO/FRH/WHD/98.16. Online. Available: http://www.who.int/reproductive-health/publications/WHD_98_16_gender_and_health_techni-cal_paper/WHD_98_16_abstract.en.html

Further reading

Schofield T, Connell RW, Walker L et al 2000 Understanding men's health and illness: a gender-relations approach to policy, research, and practice. Journal of American College Health 48: 247–256

Resources

Health professionals can use any of the public health sites referenced above as resources for their male patients/clients who want to know more about men's health and/or specific male conditions. Comparable sites for North America are the US Department of Health and Human Services: National Institutes of Health websites http://www.nih.gov/ with specific content on men's health at http://health.nih.gov/search.asp/25

Acknowledgements

I am grateful to the following colleagues for their comments and advice, which have greatly helped in shaping the manuscript.

Dr Murray Drummond
Senior Lecturer, School of Health Sciences, University of South Australia, Adelaide, Australia
Specialising in masculinity and men's body image

Kevin Rouse
Lecturer, School of Health Sciences, School of Nursing University of South Australia, Adelaide, Australia
Specialising in study of mental health and mental illness

Carol Kennedy
Senior Education Officer, Health Promotion, Drug and Alcohol Services Council, Adelaide, Australia
Specialising in primary health care

Dr Russell Waddell
Clinic manager, Sexually Transmitted Disease Services and Consultant in infectious disease, Royal Adelaide Hospital, Adelaide, Australia

Roger Levi
Clinical Nurse Specialist/Lecturer, School of Nursing, University of South Australia, Adelaide, Australia
Specialising in aged care

Chapter **1**

Sex, gender and health status

CHAPTER CONTENTS

MEN, MASCULINITY AND HEALTH

Sex and gender

Within the health literature the term sex is often used interchangeably with that of gender. However it is useful, for analytical purposes, to hold an understanding that the former relates to biology (male/female) and the latter to sexuality and social roles (masculine/feminine). Both sex and gender are relevant to understanding health and illness. A common point advanced in men's health literature is that statistically women outlive men and this suggests that there is a biological basis for health inequality. The study of men's health should extend beyond this simple statistical premise and explore the implications of men's lived experience vis-à-vis health problems, information seeking, ageing and other social circumstances that are determinants of health status. For example, men's valuing of longevity may be quite different from that of women. Men may not want longevity if it means life without being able to do masculine things or living without their spouse/partner. There are many quality of life issues for men whose partners have died. Widowed men generally have poorer health status than their female counterparts. A partial explanation for this phenomenon is that men generally lack self care skills, have less access to social supports and smaller social networks (Byrne et al 1999). These factors, when combined with living alone, have a negative effect on men's sense of wellbeing (Stewart 2001).

Researching masculinity

Masculinity is a complex concept and one that researchers and authors have tried to define for decades. Being able to define masculinity is thought to be a basis for explaining and predicting male behaviour. Connell (1995), a leading researcher on the topic, conducted a comprehensive review of various research methods employed in the last 60 years and concluded that there were substantial problems with all approaches to generalising about masculinity.

In summarising his review Connell asserted that:

- There is no single account of masculinity; instead, multiple masculinities exist.
- In recognising different types of masculinity (stereotyping) Connell (1995, p. 38) states: 'we must not take them as fixed categories' they change through time and are actively constructed in social life.
- Connell (1995, p. 37) asserts that: 'there is gender politics within masculinity' and 'to recognise diversity in masculinities is not enough. We must also recognise the *relations* between the different kinds of masculinity: *relations* of alliance, dominance and subordination.'
- Importantly, masculinity can be studied using a 'gender relations approach'. Gender relations refer to relations between men and women and relations between men and other men. The relationship is underpinned by the knowledge that masculinities are configurations of social practice such as

stereotypical gender roles (breadwinner = male role and home maker and child raiser = female role). Other configurations of stereotypical behaviour include power relations between men (e.g. oppressive action by men against homosexuals).

The last bullet point guides the reader towards an understanding that hegemony exists among men. Hegemony is the domination of one class over others, achieved by a combination of political and ideological means. Aside from the oppression of homosexuals there are other more subtle examples of men's power over men. Young men may be deterred from taking up nursing as a career because it would be seen as an attempt to adopt a traditionally female role. Connell (1995, p. 27) notes that those men who worked hard for sex role change in the early 1970s were unable to make effective resistance in the 1980s because of the 'ideologues' (other men) who rejected their ideas as a form of 'softness'. This softness was an affront to their masculinity.

Gender and health

Women have become more informed about their health and the health of others through recent socialisation. Soon after the industrial revolution women within working class families were educated about cleanliness, nutrition and the importance of reducing the use of alcohol consumption among their men folk. The impetus for this education came from the captains of industry who sought to secure a reliable and healthy workforce to service and run machinery. Since that time women have been expected to be knowledgeable about health and health issues within the family, and consequently they have amassed a variety of skills and opinions about the health of the children and spouse/partner. Women's link with nursing skills and health knowledge has become so strong that these items are often assumed to be a natural trait of females. Women have also become the main nexus between healthcare providers (doctors, nurses, organisations/special foundations) and the family. Women are best at knowing when their child is ill and keeping information about their family's health. For example, it is most often the mother that brings a child to the doctor and it is not unusual for men to turn to their wives during a health interview to ask for or confirm details about their own health history. This social history correlates well with the development of traditional gender roles, where men are perceived as masculine through activities associated with breadwinning and women are perceived as feminine through their homemaking, child raising and nursing qualities. Over generations these stereotypical social roles have come to be appreciated as natural or innate phenomena. Importantly, gender role images and discourse are constantly called upon by the media and advertising and have the effect of reinforcing these stereotypes (Gordon et al 1999).

Men's health

The emergence of 'men's health' has highlighted that men need to become knowledgeable about their bodies and need to be more proactive in accessing health services in a timely manner rather than let their problems develop to a point where the result of inaction is serious morbidity and even death. There are, however, several barriers to men achieving better health. First, it cannot be assumed that men can improve their health status by simply mimicking the approaches used by the women's health movement. Mimicking would be ineffective because the reasons for health inequalities differ between men and women. Secondly, although screening for general conditions such as hypertension, diabetes and glaucoma are effective in reducing morbidity, screening for male specific cancers has not yet been perfected. For example, although it has been shown that screening for breast cancer results in earlier diagnosis, earlier treatment and better health outcomes the same cannot be said when screening for prostate cancers (see section on 'Debates on screening' in Chapter 2). Thirdly, the literature is replete with comment concerning men's lack of help-seeking behaviour, their stoic attitude and unwillingness to communicate issues and fears; the inference being that these behaviours are identifiers of being masculine. Even though primary health activities targeting men are well subscribed to, efforts to effect long term changes in these stereotypical perceptions of what it is to be manly and what is unmanly will be more difficult to achieve (Arnot et al 1999).

Irrespective of the barrier or potential barriers there needs to be a clearer understanding of the *relationship* between masculinity and gender roles if progress towards improving men's health and well-being is to be consistent and sustainable. Those wanting to delve further into the concept of 'gender relations', need only enter 'gender and relations', as key words, in their library catalogue to find a large number of topics (sport, violence and work etc.) using this approach to exploring men and health.

Key points

- Gender is not something we are, but something we do through social interaction
- Gender is culturally determined
- Gender roles change over time
- Gender is regarded as a social determinant of health. *NSW Department of Health (2000)*

Health differentials

Sex differences in health status

Men's health issues are often based on an understanding that:

- there are *conditions* that affect only men (e.g. undescended testis)
- there are *diseases* that affect only men (testicular and prostate cancer)
- although diseases can affect both sexes some have higher rates of *mortality* or premature mortality for men (e.g. coronary heart disease).

Gender differences in health status

Men's health issues arise out of notions of what it is to be masculine.

- There are *social practices* and behaviours linked to masculinity which predispose men to health problems/injury (e.g. the habitual use of alcohol, risk taking and violence).
- Issues arise out of *society's expectations* of maleness (homophobia).
- There are unique *biological actions* relating only to the function of the male body (e.g. penile erection/impotence and ejaculation/premature ejaculation).
- There are unique *life experiences* relating only to the male psyche (e.g. fatherhood and access rights to children after spousal/partner separation).
- Issues arise out of society's expectation of *rights of passage* from boyhood to manhood.
- There are *religious affiliations* that guide men's cultural practices (e.g. circumcision, values and beliefs about men's role in society and their relationship to women).

- There are assertions that *male spirituality* is lacking in modern society.

SEX AND STATISTICS

Mortality

Death rates for both sexes declined throughout the twentieth century, though rates for males were consistently higher than rates for females. However, between 1971 and 2001 death rates for all males fell by 17% and those for all females by 5%. Mortality rates for those aged 55–64 years have also reduced considerably, falling by almost half for men and by more than a third for women.

Rising standards of living, the changing occupational structure and developments in medical technology and health practice help to explain this decline in death rates (National Statistics website). The reduction in the mortality gap between the sexes has also been attributed to:

- a decline in motor vehicle accident deaths among young men
- a decline in ischaemic heart disease among older men
- an increase in lung cancer among older women. (Australian Bureau of Statistics 2001).

Table 1.1 shows that for every 100 female deaths there are a greater number of male deaths across every age group except for the > 65 years age group. Women have a higher ratio of deaths in the over 65 years age group because a larger proportion of men have died under 65 years. Women over 65 years have higher rates of morbidity because they live with health problems for a longer period.

Table 1.1   Ratio of deaths by sex in the US (US Census Bureau 2001)

Life years	Male:female
1–4	130:100
5–14	158:100
15–24	315:100
25–44	229:100
45–64	162:100
65+	85:100

Improvement in life expectancy

Life expectancy has improved for both sexes yet men continue to have a shorter life. In the early 1900s, for richer countries around the world, the gap between female and male life expectancy was 2–3 years. By 1999, women were living on average 7–8 years more than men in those same countries (WHO 2000). Since 1981 life expectancy at birth has increased by 6 years for males and 4 years for females. In Australia a boy born between 1999 and 2001 could expect to live 77.0 years, while a girl could expect to live 82.4 years. Table 1.2 shows similar gaps in life expectancy for other industrialised nations over a similar time period.

MAJOR CAUSES OF DEATH

The identification of the leading causes of male death will help the health professional determine where health funding should be allocated to reduce the burden of disease for the individual and the nation. Although the social determinants of health (e.g. wealth, income and social privilege) have been in men's favour, males have a higher mortality rate for all 15 leading causes of death (Mathers et al 1999). In recent years cancer has overtaken ischaemic heart disease (IHD) as the leading cause of death for both men and women. This has been the result of the long term downward trend in the standardised death rate for IHD.

In England and Wales, the three main causes of death in men of all ages are IHD, stroke and lung cancer. Over the past four decades

Table 1.2   International comparison: life expectancy (years) at birth (Australian Bureau of Statistics 2002)

	Males	Females	Sex differential (years)
Japan	78	85	7
Switzerland	77	83	6
Hong Kong	77	82	5
Australia	77	82	5
Sweden	77	82	5
New Zealand	76	81	5
United Kingdom	75	80	5
United States of America	74	80	6

these diseases, when combined, accounted for 47% of all adult male deaths. Whilst there are many risk factors contributing to this trilogy of death, cigarette smoking has been found as the most common and salient risk factor (Brock & Griffiths 2003). Whilst cessation of smoking reduces the risk of IHD within a short time, the latency period for lung cancer is at least 20 years.

Cancers

Over 200 different types of cancer exist with four – breast, lung, large bowel and prostate – accounting for more than half of all new cases.

Sex difference in cancer sites

Nurses should be aware of the major cancer sites for men so that they can focus their knowledge on screening practices, diagnostic methods, treatment options and rehabilitation programmes. Table 1.3 shows the risks for the main types of cancer diagnosis in both men and women.

What are the major types of cancers affecting men?

The 10 most common cancers among males in the United Kingdom are listed in Table 1.4.

Lung cancer, once the commonest form of cancer in men, has been overtaken by prostate cancer for the first time ever. This is partly attributed to a reduction in the number of men smoking tobacco and partly due to an increase in male lifespan, where age is a prominent risk factor for prostate cancer. Information on screening practices for prostate and colorectal cancers appear later in this handbook

Table 1.3   Risk of being diagnosed with cancer over a lifetime, England and Wales (*Cancer Research UK*)

Site women	Life time risk	Site men	Life time risk
Breast	1 in 9	Prostate	1 in 14
Colorectal	1 in 20	Lung cancer	1 in 13
Lung cancer	1 in 23	Colorectal	1 in 18
Ovary	1 in 48	Bladder	1 in 30

Table 1.4   10 most common cancers among UK *males* (Cancer Research UK)

Site	Percentage of all cancers
Prostate	19%
Lung	18%
Colorectal	14%
Bladder	7%
Stomach	5%
Head and neck	4%
Non-Hodgkins's lymphoma	4%
Oesophagus	3%
Leukaemia	3%
Kidney	3%
Other	20%

Do male cancer rates differ between countries?

There are three basic reasons why male cancer rates differ between countries. First, the cancer rate in the general population is higher in some countries (e.g. colon cancer is low among Greek and African males relative to those in the UK, Australia and USA). Secondly, there are social factors which predispose males to particular types of cancer (e.g. skin cancer). Thirdly, there are cancer sites specific to males (e.g. prostate and testes) that differ between countries. Unravelling why these differences arise continues to be a major scientific task. Examples of the points just made are outlined below.

Colon cancer
The rates are higher in industrialised countries with an incidence of approximately 50 per 100 000 people in North America and northern and western Europe. Yet some African and Asian countries have rates as low as 1 per 100 000. A variety of studies indicate that the cause of this cancer depends on complex interactions between inherited susceptibility and environmental factors. This complexity makes it difficult to find evidence to use in support of any one primary prevention measure. However, diet has been identified as a key environmental factor. A strong positive correlation exists between higher rates of colon cancer and populations with high total fat intakes. On average, fat comprises 40%–45% of total caloric intake in most Western countries. Conversely, in populations where fat accounts for only 10% of dietary calories, the risk of colon

cancer is low (National Cancer Institute). This suggests that men need to reduce their total fat intake substantially. Screening for colon cancer is another modifiable lifestyle behaviour that all men should adopt. Both the United Kingdom and the United States have launched national campaigns to educate all persons over 50 years in the importance of being screened for colon cancer.

Skin cancer

This affects more men than women and there are substantial differences between countries. In countries where ultraviolet (UV) radiation reaches extreme levels there is a higher rate of most types of skin cancers. Men who are required to work outside require education and regulations regarding the use of clothing and eye wear to protect against UV rays. In Australia, 315 000 cases of non-melanoma skin cancers were diagnosed in 2001. More men than women appear to develop the cancer (NHMRC 2002). At least 850 Australians die each year from melanoma (Staples et al 1998). In the UK melanoma is a serious health issue because many people notice but do not report the lesion. Mackie et al (2002) evaluated the time taken between people first observing a worrying pigmented skin lesion and consulting their GP. Of the 162 people in the study only 67% (109) of patients attended their GP within 3 months of noticing a lesion, 25% (40) attended GPs between 3 and 12 months, and 8% (13) waited longer. However, a comparison with 1986 data showed a reduction in delays in reporting and lessening of tumour thickness at diagnosis (significance of $P < 0.001$) providing strong evidence that public education is effective.

Do male cancer rates differ between races?

The incidence of some cancers differs markedly between races; testicular and prostate cancer are the most striking examples.

Testicular cancer

The exact cause of **testicular cancer** is unknown. The clinical evidence suggests that congenital, environmental and genetic factors play an important role. Testicular cancer develops from the primordial germ cells within the testes. There are 3 main factors that may interfere with the normal development of the germ cell:

- an undescended testicle (cryptorchidism)
- exposure to chemical carcinogenesis
- a genetic predisposition.

Data indicates that about one third of patients with germ cell testicular tumours were genetically predisposed to the disease and the marked variation in incidence between racial groups is also indicative that genetics is a factor.

The incidence of testicular cancer has doubled in the US over the past 70 years and a similar trend is evident in Demark. The American Cancer Society (2005) estimates that, in the year 2005, there will be 8010 new cases of testicular cancer in the US and approximately 390 men will die of the disease. In England 5466 of hospital consultant episodes were recorded as malignant neoplasm of testis between 2002 and 2003 (Department of Health 2004).

There is no reliable data on the incidence of testicular cancer among native South Africans but it is known that the incidence of the disease is rare in this population. The incidence of this cancer also remains low among African Americans. However, it is much more common among white Americans and those Americans of mixed race. The lifetime probability of developing cancer of the testes is 0.2% (or 1 in 500) for a white male in the US. The risk of Caucasian Americans getting testicular cancer is more than five times that of African Americans and more than double that of Asian American men. Testicular cancer is also a rare occurrence among the native Japanese population resident in the United States.

Prostate cancer

The vast majority of research concerning race and **prostate cancer** emanates from the US with an emphasis on the African American population because there is a higher incidence of the disease in this group. Much of the US research findings are transferable to the African population resident in the UK:

- A longitudinal study, using 77 700 records between 1993 and 1994 revealed that mean prostate specific antigen (PSA) values differ significantly between black and white Americans (De Antoni et al 1996). Several studies have shown that African American men have higher PSA levels on average than Caucasian Americans, even after adjustment for patients' age and prostate volume (Abdalla et al 1998). The clinical significance of race-specific PSA reference ranges has yet to be determined.
- African American males have a higher incidence and higher mortality rates and present with higher stage and grade of prostate cancer than other racial groups in the US.

- Freeman et al (1997) found that even after adjusting for the stage of cancer development at presentation, African Americans had a significantly higher burden of high histologic prostate cancer than Caucasian Americans.
- The survival disadvantage of black men with local stage cancer is due in part to a propensity for the development of less differentiated and more aggressive malignancies (Fowler et al 2000).
- Although there is evidence suggesting that African Americans have more aggressive prostate cancer, the role of race as a factor in outcome is significantly decreased if the cancer is diagnosed and treated early enough (Powell et al 2004).

Race and access to health

Early research suggested that African Americans present with more advanced prostate cancer and this goes some way to explaining a lower survival rate among this group of men (Roach et al 1992). Elsewhere in the literature, barriers to accessing care, the quality of care received, and the impact of co-morbid conditions are also cited as possible explanations for the lower survival reported for African Americans. However, Hart et al (1999) concluded that if African American males with early-stage prostate cancer receive timely radiotherapy they can expect similar biochemical disease-free survival rates to those seen in Caucasian males with the same treatment. By studying men who had equal access to the same health care system of the Department of Defense, Johnstone et al (2002) were able to show that African American race was not associated with a consistently negative prognosis in patients treated with definitive radiation therapy for prostate cancer. The conclusion was that race appeared to confer a negative prognosis only in patients with advanced disease at presentation. Provided there is equal access to health care, race does not appear to adversely affect bio-chemical disease-free survival in males treated for early-stage prostate cancer.

Heart disease

Men develop coronary heart disease (CHD) earlier than women partly because women have substantial protection in the form of premenopausal hormones and partly because men's lifestyle habits (e.g. smoking, dietary intake of animal fats) are strongly linked to

CHD. As a consequence, men aged 45–54 years have a death rate of 100/100 000 per year and women for the same age group have a rate of only 20/100 000. An alternative statistic, supplied by the British Heart Foundation (2002), is that men run a 2% risk of having a myocardial infarction (MI) before the age of 60 years (1 in 50 men) whereas women have only half that risk (1 in 100).

The risk of dying from an MI has roughly halved from what it was in 1980. However, UK death rates from coronary heart disease continue to be among the highest in the world, accounting for 23% of premature deaths in men and 14% in women. This is because the UK has high levels of standard risk factors with relatively low levels of interventions against these risks (Poulter 2003).

Angina pectoris affects 2–3% of the population, equating to an estimated 2.21 million people in the UK. The number of males consulting their GP for angina pectoris in 2002 was estimated at 327 000 (307 000 for women). There were also 78 300 male and 59 200 female discharges from hospital for the principal diagnosis of angina pectoris or unstable angina (Stewart et al 2003).

Nurses and other health professionals should focus on assessing men with angina for:

- financial and quality of life issues because of the debilitating nature of this condition
- psychological changes linked to unemployment or under-employment as a consequence of debilitating symptoms.

A sense of diminished self-worth leading to depression is common in these circumstances.

HEALTH CONCERNS OF ADULTS

For nurses intending to work in primary health, it is useful to know of the strong correlation between what health researchers identify as major health issues and what individuals believe are the main concerns. However, individuals' knowledge of the risks to their health does not always translate into healthier behaviours.

What are the major health concerns in the UK, US and Australia?

- Cigarette smoking
- Alcohol related mortality
- Road accidents

- Suicide
- Home and work-related accidents
- Drug-related poisoning
- Sexually transmitted diseases.

Readers can refer to the section on health promotion to view national strategies to correct these health problems.

SOCIAL DETERMINANTS OF HEALTH

The term 'social determinants of health' has developed as a means of establishing a link between social forces and the health status of individuals and communities. For example:

- research dating back over 100 years indicates that a fragmentation of society positively influences suicide rates among men (Whitley et al 1999);
- health services are concentrated in geographical areas where they are needed least (those with access to wealth and income usually have better health).

Nurses working in communities and with those who are socially disadvantaged will understand at first hand that social as well as physical factors strongly influence health status and outcomes. Marmot (1999) refers to social factors such as employment status, transport, housing, literacy, patterns of social relationships, social exclusion, food, addictive behaviour, early childhood environment and work environment as being key elements in socially determining health.

Nursing issues

An exemplar of a social determinant of health: the disadvantaged male
Obtaining a timely diagnosis for advanced prostate cancer represents a major health problem for low-income men. The study by Bennett et al (1998) suggests that opportunities vary for early detection of prostate cancer for low-income African and Caucastian American men because of financial, cultural and social factors.

Nursing issues—cont'd

Bennett et al found that African American men were:

- almost twice as likely to present with stage D prostate cancer as their Caucasian counterparts (49.5% v 35.9%; $P < 0.05$)
- significantly more likely to have literacy levels less than sixth grade (52.3% v 8.7%; $P < 0.001$).

Low literacy is a significant barrier to the diagnosis of early-stage prostate cancer among low-income men of African and Caucasian origin.

Implications for nursing practice

- Aim to improve the frequency of diagnosis of early-stage cancer among high risk groups.
- Seek out culturally sensitive information on urinary symptoms for men.
- Develop low-literacy educational materials with the aim of improving men's awareness of prostate cancer (Bennett et al 1998).

Poverty

Poverty often limits access to appropriate medical services and can limit treatment options for men and their families. The positive correlation between social deprivation and mortality and morbidity is well established in most developed countries (Townsend & Davidson 1982, Burdess 1996):

- One in 5 men live in poverty (Oxfam 2003).
- Mortality tends to be higher in people living in poor areas irrespective of their socioeconomic position.
- Minority ethnic groups in the UK are often more vulnerable to poverty.
- People in the lower socioeconomic groups make considerably less use of illness prevention and health promotional services than those higher up.
- There is evidence to show that drug companies neglect research into diseases affecting the poor.
- 'The burden of psychiatric morbidity is disproportionately borne by the socially and culturally disadvantaged. Men feature prominently in this social group' (Pilgrim & Rogers 1993; p. 13).

Nursing issues

Implications for nursing practice
Although their level of wealth and income are sensitive issues for most men, nurses play an important role when they explore these factors. Nurses:

- should gain an understanding of a man's access to resources that contribute to better health (do they have enough money to make healthier choices?)
- can determine the likelihood of adherence to treatment by asking if the man has enough money to pay for prescribed drugs or treatments
- need to be able to identify issues with men who are unable to work because of disability, illness, injury
- can provide valuable support for men who have concerns about their ability to pay for family health care

Nurses should explore sociological concepts such as the 'poverty trap' and effects of long term unemployment to provide insight and empathy. This approach will reduce the likelihood of making value laden and stereotypical judgements about patients from lower socio-economic groups.

Divorce

Separation and divorce are stressful for all parties but men and women have different responses and coping mechanisms. Research has shown that women are more likely to seek help from friends, religious counsel, marriage guidance organisations, doctors and pharmacists. Men may have more extreme responses to separation and divorce than their partners, affecting their ability to work and to relate to others. A British study revealed that 24% of men had 'severe' mental health problems and 9% experienced new and 'very severe' mental health problems linked to divorce (Rogers 1996). Although alcohol is often used by men to overcome emotional problems following relationship breakdown, alcohol has also been recognised as a contributing factor in 1 in 3 divorces in the UK.

Nurses can play a key role in assessing and gaining an understanding of men's emotional and physiological reactions to separation and divorce.

Men reactions may be more extreme because:
- Men are less dissatisfied with the relationship
- They had a preference not to separate
- Lack of awareness of the issues
- Ignorance of the wife's views on separation
- They were being left and felt rejected.

Effects of separation and divorce on wellbeing

- Sleeplessness
- Headaches
- Poor memory and concentration
- Crying
- Lethargy
- Poor appetite
- Tight muscles.

Factors for nurses to consider when making a risk assessment

- Men's reactions (listed above) emphasise the need for nurse counsellors.
- The effects on wellbeing (listed above) may affect men's safety (workplace).
- Many men use antidepressants, tranquillisers or sleeping tablets (affecting driving and work).
- Emotional reactions can trigger physical health problems (gastric ulcers).
- Men may use alcohol to ease emotional pain (alcohol use could have contributed to separation and may affect outcomes of child custody claims).

Nursing interviews

Nurses who interview men who are separating or divorcing need to identify issues that cause distress and highlight resources that support adjustment to divorce. Key stressors include:

- decline in standard of living (financial hardship when the original family income becomes split across two households)
- losing friends (reductions in social network size caused by his friend/her friend delineation)

- moving residence (the stress of moving and large declines in per capita income reduces options for residence)
- people who hold negative attitudes towards divorce.

Adjustment to divorce

Understanding how and when adjustment to divorce takes place may assist the nurse in determining when supportive resources are most needed. Most studies have used broad indicators of general adjustment.

- psychological distress
- self-reported health
- extent of substance use.

These three items, though indicative of stress, have been found to be relatively poor predictors of the extent of adjustment to divorce, except among those men not employed (Wang & Amato 2000). Several studies show that level of education, employment and income are positively related to psychological adjustment among divorced individuals. Relatively few studies have explored the role of race in moderating divorce effects on individuals.

Periods of mourning for relationship loss

Although both the partner who leaves and the partner who is left experience emotional pain and stress, the timing of the distress and recovery differs, the assumption being that the spouses who initiate divorce have completed all or most of their mourning by the time the physical separation and legal divorce occur. Conversely, those who resisted the divorce are likely to experience most of their mourning after these events. As men are much less likely to have initiated the divorce, have fewer confidants and have usually lost custody of their children, it would seem as though they might be more negatively affected. However, Wang and Amato (2000), using a longitudinal approach and telephone interviews with 2033 Americans, found little evidence to show that the predictors of adjustment operated differently for women and men. Other studies also show that gender was not associated with general divorce adjustment or evaluations of life (Wang & Amato 2000). Those best adjusted tended to be those who initiated the divorce and/or who were in a new relationship.

Imprisonment

For most of the men imprisoned in the UK their term is for less than 6 months. Nevertheless, at any one time approximately 65 000 people are held in one of 135 prisons in England and Wales. The average male population in 2002 was 66 480 (female 4300). A high proportion of prisoners come from socially excluded sections of our community, and a recent survey showed that 90% of those entering prison had a mental health or substance misuse problem (HMPS 2003). National data on the health status of Australian prisoners is not available (AIHW 2002).

In the UK *Prison Health* is a partnership between the Prison Service and the Department of Health working to improve the standard of health care in prisons. Their aim is to provide prisoners with access to the same quality and range of health care services as the general public receives from the NHS (DOH 2003).

Prisoners are likely to have poor health status related to:

- Communicable diseases (e.g. hepatitis C and B)
- HIV infection
- Injecting illicit drugs
- Heavy smoking
- Consuming harmful/hazardous amounts of alcohol (prior to imprisonment)
- Depression
- Committing self-harm
- Suicide (mostly by hanging).

Policy change

The Home Secretary and the Secretary of State for Health agreed that funding responsibility for prison health services in England is to be transferred from the Home Office to the Department of Health. This responsibility took effect from April 2003. This is the first step in a process over the next 5 years which will see prison health become part of the NHS.

Nursing issues

Social prejudice against minority groups and the socially disadvantaged is common. Laying blame on those with health problems (victim blaming) is also a problematic behaviour. Nurses can rise above this reactive stance by developing a clearer understanding of the factors that contribute to poor living and working conditions and impose severe restrictions on an individual's ability to choose a healthier life style.
Spend some time considering the following:

- What are the major social determinants on health?
- What are the major economic determinants on health?
- What control does the disadvantage have over the person's lifestyle?
- What local and national policies support equitable access and quality of services?
- What local and national resources are available to assist in making healthier choices easier for the disadvantaged?
- How does a nursing code of ethics guide your practice in terms of caring for the socially disadvantaged?

MENTAL HEALTH

Although historically women have more mental health problems than men, this phenomenon has been attributed to social construction of mental illness by male experts (women have more classifications of mental illness and are more likely to receive a formal diagnosis). The gender difference in lifetime prevalence is 3:1 (male : female). A landmark survey conducted in the US in the mid 1980s, The Epidemiological Catchment Area study, determined that 20% of both males and females aged 18 years and over had a 'mental disorder' (Robins & Regier 1991). However, a distinct sex pattern has been noted in diagnosis; men have much higher rates of alcohol abuse and anti-social personality traits whilst women have higher rates of depression, obsessive-compulsive disorder and somatisation (NHMRC 1996).

Poverty

The burden of psychiatric morbidity is disproportionately borne by the socially and culturally disadvantaged and men feature prominently in this social group (Pilgrim & Rogers 1993, p. 13).

Boys

A review of studies in England, the US, Australia, New Zealand and Canada revealed that boys have a higher incidence of mental disorder and maladjustment (Sawyer 1996). Whilst girls had more phobias and separation anxiety, boys were found to have more depression, attention deficit disorders, oppositional and conduct disorders. Boys more frequently experience a wide range of severe mental health disabilities, such as autism.

Service use

The National Health and Medical Research Council (NHMRC) of Australia (1996) reported that although there is little variance in overall prevalence in mental disorder between males and females, there is a difference in service utilisation. 73% of private services, funded by Medicare, were used by females. In contrast, boys more frequently attended public mental health services.

Nursing issues

For nurses who have not specialised in mental health the assessment and management of a person with an aberrant behaviour is likely to present some challenges. Consider:

● How do you react upon hearing that your patient has a mental health diagnosis?

Spend some time considering these findings:

● The unpredictable or unusual behaviour exhibited by patients can evoke a sense of fear in nurses. Who would you seek out to develop strategies to cope with this?
● Fear is often associated with a lack of knowledge about mental health problems and fear may be evoked by an adherence to commonly held myths. What do you believe are myths about mental health that need dispelling?

Nursing issues—cont'd

- People with a mental health problem are perceived as being more likely to commit acts of violence than other members of a community. In reality, apart from a very narrow range of diagnosis (paranoid schizophrenia), people with a mental health problem are less likely to be violent. Does this information surprise you? Where would you seek more information on why violence occurs between nurses and patients with a mental health problem?
- If you have concerns about caring for people with mental health problems, what strategies would you use to overcome those concerns?

Mental health assessment

Nurses who work in community settings or in general hospitals are likely to encounter people who have a mental disorder. As such, it is important for all nurses to be able to make an objective assessment of patients who they believe are displaying inappropriate behaviours. For those nurses who do not have mental health as a specialty in their practice, the task of making a mental health assessment can be challenging. The mnemonic ABC, APC, described below, is a guide to making a systematic assessment for the purpose of documentation in case notes and as a basis for referral to specialist psychiatric evaluation and care (Laws & Rouse 1996).

Structuring a mental state assessment

The mnemonic ABC, APC will assist in documenting your observations in an objective manner and as such will assist in writing a referral to a member of the mental health liaison team:

- **Appearance** (physical characteristics, describe manner of dress, posture, hygiene)
- **Behaviour** (gestures, unusual movements, gait, body language)
- **Conversation** (quantity of talk, volume of talk, rhythm of speech, articulation of sounds, e.g. slurring)

- **Affect** (report your own as well as the patients' perceptions of their mood and emotions)
- **Perception** (note the clients' experience of their world from what they state, e.g. 'they are trying to kill me', 'no one cares about me')
- **Cognition** (use questioning to assess recollections, i.e. short term/long term memory, questions about time and place). (*Adapted from Laws & Rouse 1996*)

An alternative and more detailed form of mental health assessment can be found in Teifion (1997).

Diagnosis of mental health disorders

The *Diagnostic and Statistical Manual of Mental Disorders* (DSM), published by the American Psychiatric Association (1989), is a guide to the classification and diagnosis of mental disorders. This manual is often used in the UK, along with other guidelines for the diagnosis of mental illness (see NHS Direct website, http://www.nhsdirect.nhs.uk/en.asp? TopicID-57&AreaID-3509&LinkID-2584). The most up-to-date version is the fourth edition, DSM-IV-TR, published in 2000.

Nursing issues

Spend some time considering the following:

- What is the value of using a systematic process for assessing the mental health status of your patients?
- How would you document your assessment of a patient who is behaving inappropriately?
- Who would you choose to validate your mental health assessment findings?
- What resources do you have to assist you in the patient's care?
- How would you locate information pertaining to psychiatric medication?
- What is your organisation's policy on management of aggressive patients?

Suicide

Suicide is a complex phenomenon to study because of the variability in circumstances and psychology of people taking their own lives. The focus is not only on identifying those at risk and finding effective management strategies, but also towards the survivors (friends, relatives, acquaintances) who are left asking 'why did this happen'?

Australia

Whilst incidence of suicide rate was less than 2% of all deaths in 1998, this equated to 2683 people taking their own lives that year. Of these, 2150 were male suicides. For every completed suicide there are 30 attempts recorded. Men tend to be more successful because of the means used (e.g. firearms, hanging, carbon monoxide, poison). Whilst the focus has been on teenage suicides, these account for only 16.6% of total suicides. The rate for men aged 24–44 (middle age) has increased by 44% since 1979. For women of 24–44 years the suicide rates are 25% less. The rate of suicide for men over 70 is also growing (ABS 2000). Australian suicide rates for 15–24 and 25–34 year old males rose between 1964 and 1997. Comparatively, female rates showed no significant change in that time. International comparisons have found that whereas Australian youth suicide rates are relatively high, it is not the same for men in the older age groups. Although youth is an appropriate priority group for assessment and intervention strategies, Cantor et al (1999) contend that the age range should be extended to include 25–34 year olds.

America

On average, 85 Americans die from suicide each day. Although more females attempt suicide, males are at least 4 times more likely to die from suicide. Firearms account for 59% of all suicides in the US. Over half a million Americans are treated annually for attempted suicide (Office of the Surgeon General 1999).

UK

There are around 5000 suicides every year in the UK with 75% of suicides carried out by males. In the 25–44 age range, men are almost four times more likely than women to kill themselves.

Although there has been a 6% decrease in the overall suicide rate since 1991, the number of young males who commit suicide each year in the UK has doubled over the last ten years. Non-fatal acts of self harm are estimated at 142 000 cases each year in England and Wales (NHS 2005). There is a national suicide prevention strategy, annual report available through the Department of Health (2005) website.

DoH Goals (UK)

The HDA website (http://www.hda-online.org.uk/hdt/1202/analysis.html) outlines the six goals and three major plans for action to prevent suicide:

- To reduce the risk of self harm among high risk groups, including young men
- To promote mental wellbeing in the wider population
- To reduce the availability and lethal effects of suicide methods
- To improve the reporting of suicidal behaviour in the media
- To promote research on suicide and its prevention
- To improve the monitoring of progress towards the national suicide prevention target (to cut suicides by 20% by 2010)

(Department of Health National Institute for Mental Health in England 2005).

Nursing issues

Nurses have viewed patients who repeatedly attempt suicide or self harm as less than deserving of care. Conversely, people with strokes and myocardial infarctions deserve care because their condition is perceived to be largely out of their control.

Spend some time discussing this issue with colleagues and other health professionals so that you can resolve this issue and consider factors such as codes of ethics, cost of care, benefits of treating all patients equally.

Also identify what resources are available in your region or health service to support these patients in reducing the incidence and severity of self harm

Detecting suicidal ideation

Nurse might be able to detect and refer those at risk of attempting suicide to specialist health services if they were aware of the risk factors. However, measures to screen those individuals at greatest risk lack precision. It is because screening is not effective that suicide prevention efforts need to take a broad approach (e.g. emergency helplines and clinical care for those identified as struggling with suicidal ideation).

Suicide risk factors

- Previous suicide attempt
- Mental disorder
- Depression and bipolar disorder
- Co-occurring alcohol and substance abuse
- Family history of suicide
- Discourse signifying hopelessness
- Impulsive and/or agitated tendencies
- Physical illness
- Ease of access to firearms
- Sexually abused as a child
- Marital discord/separation from spouse/partner and children
- Separation from children
- Unemployment. (Office of the Surgeon General 1999)

NB. Unemployment should be included as a risk factor for men because it impacts on their sense of self-worth more so than on women. The role of breadwinner is a key component of self-identify for men.

Confirming suicidal ideation

When confronted with someone who intimates suicide the nurse can:

- Ask the direct question 'Do you intend to kill yourself?'
- Ask 'Do you have a plan?'
- Ask 'What method would you use?'
- Ask 'Is there a time and place and why have you chosen those?'
- Interview the patient to identify if risk factors are present.

This information should be documented when referring the person to a mental health specialist.

Key points

Even if a person exhibits a large number of the risk factors associated with suicide there is currently no tool that effectively predicts which individual will follow through on plans to commit suicide.

People who self harm are likely to be seeking recognition of problems they hold rather than intending to commit suicide. In this sense self harm is a different phenomenon to those people who intend and plan, in detail, their suicide. Additionally, some people can make suicide attempts impulsively, adding to the difficulties of predicting who is most at risk.

Of those people who repeatedly self harm, there are 10% that actually carry through and commit suicide. The rationale for the progression from self harm to suicide is that in each attempt to self harm their methods become closer to lethal. Some individuals shift from self harm to a successful suicide attempt because they have changed their perception and want closure on their problems.

Cognitive behavioural therapy is thought to be as effective in managing depression as medication. Importantly, depression is a key diagnosis associated with suicidal ideation and attempted suicide.

Depression

In Britain:

* One in 10 adults suffers from depression
* Figures for men are 36–48/1000
* Figures for women are 89–96/1000. (see Health Development Agency website http://www.hda.nhs.uk/search/search results.asp? SEARCHTERMS-depression

Surveys similar to the US Epidemiological Catchment Area study (mentioned at the beginning of this mental health section) were carried out in Australia and New Zealand. The Australian study found that 6.7% of males and 14.1% of females were suffering from depression. The New Zealand study noted major depression for 3.4% of males and 7.1% of females (NHMRC 1996).

Depression in older men

The Health Development Agency (see website: http://www.hda. nhs.uk/search/search results.asp? SEARCHTERMS-depression) has provided an evidence-based briefing on depression among older people. The agency concludes that research has focused on treatments for depression rather than an understanding of the social and cultural issues that may affect the nature and extent of the problem. What is known is that:

- 70% of older people consulted their GP in the month prior to suicide.
- 33% of older people consulted their GP within a week prior to suicide.
- There is little consensus on what needs to be done.
- Screening measures do exist for older adults (Beck Depression Inventory).
- Screening is recommended above simple clinical judgement at time of consult.
- Interpersonal psychotherapy can be effective for acute episodes (e.g. grief).
- Crisis lines are available (e.g. http://www.samaritans.co.uk/) and intuitively they provide much needed support. However, their effectiveness has been systematically evaluated.
- Systematic reviews are needed to explore the nexus between ageism, social support and disability (physical, mental).

Post traumatic stress disorder

It is widely recognised that emergency health service personnel, (e.g. ambulance, fire, police), men at war, POWs and even nurses have been exposed to critical incidents (Laws 2001). A critical incident is any situation that causes strong emotional reactions that interferes with the person's ability to function at the scene or later. Signs of critical incident stress (CIS) include restlessness, irritability, excessive fatigue, sleep disturbances, anxiety, startle reactions, depression, moodiness, muscle tremors, difficulties in concentrating, nightmares, vomiting and diarrhoea. If symptoms are ignored the stress response could progress to a formal diagnosis of Post Traumatic Stress Disorder (PTSD).

How is PTSD diagnosed?

The DSM-IV (American Psychiatric Association 2000) has classified PTSD as a subtype of anxiety disorders. The WHO's ICD–10–CM (WHO) does not have a classification for PTSD. PTSD is not easily recognised because it has shared features with other mental disorders (anxiety, depression).

Which men are most affected by CIS or PTSD?

- Emergency services personnel
- War veterans (Gulf War syndrome)
- Members of the public witnessing a critical incident
- Victims of trauma (rape, torture, shootings).

An analysis of mental health disorder in men who have been to war (Second World War, Vietnam, Falklands, the Gulf War) has concluded that different wars have different effects on men's mental health.

Implications for nursing care of veterans

The effects of war persist for years and nurses can expect to find:

- A high prevalence of alcohol-related problems
- High levels of phobias (particularly Vietnam veterans)
- High level of anxiety disorders (particularly Second World War veterans)
- PTSD (45% POWs, 27% non-POWs). (O'Toole et al 1996)

The Second World War veteran population is dwindling; more recent veterans (from conflicts in Korea, the Falklands, the Gulf War) experience relatively less in terms of veteran services. Coupled to this is the insult that the Vietnam War was never officially declared and as such public recognition of their efforts has been muted. These factors contribute greatly to veterans experiencing social and general phobias (O'Toole et al 1996).

CULTURAL IDENTITIES AMONG MEN

Men are not a homogeneous group as their identity is shaped by social norms specific to their culture, life experiences and personal preferences. These factors, added to multiple forms of masculinity, make it difficult to generalise about men's health beliefs and practices. The following items exemplify the scantiness of data we hold on men and their health practices.

Ethnicity

Whilst a large number of ethnic groups have been studied in relation to their health status, the vast majority of these works address the status of women, whilst men only 'feature briefly' (Manderson & Reid 1994, Julian & Easthope 1996). Cooper et al (2000) note that there has been a less than systematic investigation of the disadvantages that may be experienced by older ethnic minority groups living in the UK and that ethnicity and age are rarely integrated in health research. There are also problems collecting and collating data on the health status of ethnic groups in some countries because data collection methods are not standardised (Mathers et al 1996). Moreover, few studies concern themselves with understanding the passing on of health practices between men and boys within ethnic groups (Laws & Bradley 2003).

Spirituality

There is a clear need to establish a mechanism to identifying the religious and spiritual needs of men. However, Clatterbaugh (1997) argues that while the feminist movement has brought women's spirituality to the fore, men have yet to find healthy and vigorous ways to do the same. The exception is the reunification of masculinity and spirituality in the form of the mytho-poetic movement (sometimes referred to as men in the woods, drum beating) headed by Robert Bly and John Rowan.

Nursings' central tenet, that of holistic care, is reflected in the large number of nursing publications linking spirituality with health (Ronaldson 1997). However, literature linking men and spirituality is sparse. Emblem and Halstead (1993) observed that most male patients were reluctant to discuss spirituality, and many male nurses expressed reservations about discussing personal issues related to spirituality. Yet there is an increasing emphasis on spirituality as a factor contributing to wellbeing and coping strategies (B 2004). Awareness that spiritual needs change with time and circumstances is prompting healthcare teams to effect accurate and timely evaluation of spiritual issues through regular assessment.

This review process is particularly relevant to those newly diagnosed with a terminal illness.

Religion

In Anderson et al's (1993) US study of patients receiving rehabilitation services, 74% indicated their religious and spiritual beliefs were important. 45% indicated not enough attention was paid to their religious or spiritual needs. Only a marginal majority of patients (54%) desired pastoral visitation. Although essentially supportive, religious faith can also have a detrimental effect on a patient's recovery. Many Jewish patients in Anderson et al's study reported concerns about being punished by God, and some Christian patients were concerned that God was unaware of their personal needs. Some responders, regardless of personal faith, were also troubled by God's failure to heal.

References

Abdalla I, Ray P, Vijayakumar S 1998 Race and serum prostate-specific antigen levels: current status and future directions. Seminars in Urologic Oncology 16(4): 207–213

American Cancer Society 2005 Overview. Testicular cancer. How many men get Testicular cancer? Online. Available: http://www.cancer.org/docroot/CRI/content/CRI 2 2 1x How Many People Get Testicular Cancer 41.asp?sitearea

American Psychiatric Association 1989 Diagnostic and statistical manual of mental disorder, 3rd edn. APA, Washington DC p 236–238

American Psychiatric Association 2000 Diagnostic and statistical manual of mental disorder, 4th edn. (DSM–IV) APA, Washington DC, p 463

Anderson JM, Anderson LJ, Felsenthal G 1993 Pastoral needs and support within an inpatient rehabilitation unit. Archives of Physical Medicine and Rehabilitation 74(6): 574–578

Arnot M, Weiner GM, David M 1999 Closing the gender gap: postwar education and social change. Blackwell, Cambridge

Australian Bureau of Statistics 2000 Suicides, Australia, 1921–1998. ABS, Canberra

Australian Bureau of Statistics 2002 Australia now. Australian social trends 2001. Health – mortality and morbidity: mortality in the 20th century. Online. Available: http://www.abs.gov.au/ausstats/abs@. nsf/0/7C1C9A5083F7DFB7CA256BCD0082556E?Open

Australian Bureau of Statistics 2004 **Deaths, Australia** 2003. Australian Bureau of Statistics Canberra. Catalogue no. 3302.0. Online. Available: www.abs.gov.au/websitedbs/C311215.nsf/0/80330B4BDEACFE2ECA256ECA000CF25E?Open

Australian Institute of Health and Welfare (AIHW) 2002 Australia's health 2002: the eighth biannual health report. Australia's Health No. 8. AIHW, Canberra

Bennet CL, Ferreira MR, Davis TC et al 1998 Relation between literacy, race and stage of presentation among low-income patients with prostate cancer. Journal of Clinical Oncology 16(9): 3101–3104

British Heart Foundation 2002 Factfiles. 11–2002: Understanding risk part II: coronary heart disease. Online. Available: www.bhf.org.uk/factfiles.

Brock AC, Griffiths C 2003 Trends in the mortality of young adults aged 15–44 in England and Wales, 1961 to 2001. Health Statistics Quarterly 19(27): 22–31

Burdess N 1996 Class and health. In: Gribich C (ed) Health in Australia, sociological concepts and issues. Prentice Hall, Sydney

Byrne GJA, Raphael B, Arnold E 1999 Alcohol consumption and psychological distress in recently widowed older men. Australian and New Zealand Journal of Psychiatry 5(33): 740–747

Cancer Research UK. CancerStats Incidence–UK. Online. Available: http://www.cancerresearchuk.org/aboutcancer/statistics/statsmisc/pdfs/cancerstats_incidence.pdf

Cantor CH, Neulinger K, De Leo D 1999 Australian suicide trends 1964–1997 – youth and beyond? Medical Journal of Australia 171: 137–141

Clatlerbaugh K 1997 Contemporary perspectives on masculinity: men, women and politics in modern society, 2nd edn. Westview Press, Boulder CO

Connell R 1995 Masculinities. Hartnolls, Bodmin

Cooper H, Arber S, Daly T et al 2000 Ethnicity, health and health behavior: a study of older groups. Health Development Agency, Leo

DeAntoni EP, Crawford ED, Oesterling JE et al 1996 Age- and race-specific reference ranges for prostate-specific antigen from a large community-based study. Urology 48(2): 234–239

Department of Health 2003 Prison health. Online. Available: www.doh.gov.uk/prisonhealth/index.htm

Department of Health 2004 Hospital episode statistics 2002–2003. Online. Available: http://www.dh.gov.uk/PublicationsAndStatistics/Statistics/HospitalEpisodeStatistics/HESFreeData/Fs/en

Department of Health National Institute for Mental Health in England 2005 National suicide prevention strategy for England: annual report on progress 2004. Online. Available: http://www.dh.gov.uk/PublicationsAnd Statistics/Publications/AnnualReports/DHAnnualReportsArticle/Fs/en?CONTENT ID-4101668&chk-ZALnoC

Emblem JD, Halstead L 1993 Spiritual needs and interventions: comparing the views of patients, nurses and chaplains. Clinical Nurse Specialist 7(4): 175–182

Fowler JE Jr, Bigler SA, Bowman G et al 2000 Race and cause specific survival with prostate cancer: influence of clinical stage, Gleason score, age and treatment. Journal of Urology 163(1): 137–142

Freeman VL, Leszczak J, Cooper RS 1997 Race and the histologic grade of prostate cancer. Prostate 30(2): 79–84

Gordan D 1999 The ethics of 'correctness' and 'inclusiveness': culture, race, and gender in the mass media. In: Gordon D, Merill J, Kittross J et al (eds) Controversies in media ethics. Longman, New York

Hart KB, Wood DP Jr, Tekyi-Mensah S et al 1999 The impact of race on biochemical disease-free survival in early-stage prostate cancer patients treated with surgery or radiation therapy. International Journal of Radiation Oncology, Biology and Physics 45(5): 1235–1238

Her Majesty's Prison Service. Health and welfare in custody. Online. Available: http://www.hmprisonservice.gov. uk/life/dynpage.asp?page=1033

Johnstone PA, Kane CJ, Sun L et al 2002 Effect of race on biochemical disease-free outcome in patients with prostate cancer treated with definitive radiation therapy in an equal-access health care system: radiation oncology report of the Department of Defense Center for Prostate Disease Research. Radiology 225(2): 420–426

Julian R, Easthope G 1996 Migrant health. In: Gribich C (ed) Health in Australia: social concepts and issues. Prentice Hall, Sydney

Laws TA 2001 Examining critical care nurses' critical incident stress after in hospital emergency cardiopulmonary resuscitation (CPR). Australian Critical Care 14(2): 76–81

Laws TA, Bradley H 2003 A comparison of health knowledge and practices transferred from men to boys within indigenous and non-indigenous Australian families. Contemporary Nurse 15(3): 249–261

Laws TA, Rouse K 1996 Mental health assessment for all nurses. Australian Nursing Journal 2(7): 32–35

Mackie RM, Bray CA, Leman JA 2003 Effect of public education aimed at early diagnosis of malignant melanoma: cohort comparison study. British Medical Journal 326(7385): 367

Manderson L, Reid F (1994) What has culture got to do with it? In: Gribich C (ed) Just health: inequality in illness, care and prevention. Churchill Livingstone, Edinburgh

Marmot M 1999 Social determinants of health. Oxford University Press, Oxford

Mathers CD, Armstrong B, Waters AM et al 1996 Identification of ethnicity and indigenous status in national health and welfare data collections. Information paper. AIHW, Canberra

Mathers CD, Sadana R, Salomon J et al 1999 Health life expectancy in 191 countries. Lancet 357(9269): 1685–1691

National Cancer Institute. CancerWeb. Prevention of colorectal cancer. 208/04731 Online. Available: http://cancerweb.ncl.ac.uk/cancernet/304731.html

National Health and Medical Research Council (NHMRC) 1996 Men and mental health. Australian Government Publishing Service. Online. Available: http://www.nhmrc.gov.au/publication/pdf/mh11.pdf

National Health and Medical Research Council (NHMRC) 2002 Australia and Europe to research HPV link to skin cancer. Press release 27 Dec 2002. Online. Available: http://www.nhmrc.gov.au/media/2002rel/hvp.htm#top

National Health Service 2005 NHS Direct online health encyclopaedia. Bipolar affective disorder. Diagnosis. Online. Available: http://www.nhsdirect.nhs.uklen.asp?Topic ID-57&AreaID-3509&LinkID-2584

National Statistics Website. Deaths: by age and sex, 1971–2021: social trends 33 Online. Available: http://www.statistics.gov.uk/

New South Wales Department of Health 2000 Gender equity in health. Better Health Centre, Gladesville, New South Wales

Office of the Surgeon General 1999 Surgeon General's report an suicide – 1999. Online. Available: http://www.menstuff.org/issues/byissue/surgeongen.html

O'Toole BI, Marshall RP, Grayson DA et al 1996 War and mental health. In: Jorm AF (ed) Men and mental health. NHMRC Australian Government Printing Service, Canberra

Oxfam 2003 The facts about poverty in the UK. Online. Available: http://www.oxfamgb.org/ukpp/poverty/thefacts.htm

Pilgrim D, Rogers A 1993 A sociology of mental illness. Open University Press, Buckingham

Poulter N 2003 Global risk of cardiovascular disease. (includes discussion). Heart (British Cardiac Society) 89 (S ii): ii2–5

Powell IJ, Banerjee M, Bianco FJ et al 2004 The effect of race/ethnicity on prostate cancer treatment outcome is conditional: a review of Wayne State University data. Journal of Urology 171(4): 1508–1512

Roach M III, Krall J, Keller JW et al 1992 The prognostic significance of race and survival from prostate cancer based on patients irradiated on Radiation Therapy Oncology Group protocols (1976–1985). International Journal of Radiation Oncology Biology and Physics 24(3): 441–449

Robins LN, Regier DA (eds) 1991 Psychiatric disorders in America: the Epidemiologic Catchment Area Study. Free Press, New York

Rogers B 1996 Separation, divorce and mental health. In: Jorm AF (ed) Men and mental health. NHMRC Australian Government Printing Service, Canberra

Ruxton S 2001 Men, masculinities and poverty. Oxfam, Oxford

Sawyer MG (1996) Childhood mental health problems. In: Jorm AF (ed) Men and mental health. NHMRC Australian Government Printing Service, Canberra

Staples MP, Marks R, Giles GG 1998 Trends in the incidence of non-melanocytic skin cancer (NMSC) treated in Australia 1985–1995: are primary prevention programs starting to have an effect? International Journal of Cancer 78: 144–148

Stewart M, Craig MacPherson K, Alexander S 2001 Promoting positive affect and diminishing loneliness of widowed seniors through a support intervention. Public Health Nursing 18(1): 54–63

Stewart S, Murphy N, Walker A et al 2003 The current cost of angina pectoris to the National Health Service in the UK. Heart 89:1–6

Teifion D 1997 ABC of mental health: mental health assessment. British Medical Journal 314(7093): 1536

Townsend P, Davidson N (1982) Inequalities in health. The Black report. Penguin, London

US Census Bureau 2001 statistical abstract of the United States (1997). Health and nutrition. Online. Available: http://www.census.gov/prod/www/statistical-abstract-us.html

Wang H, Amato PR 2000 Predictors of divorce adjustment: stressors, resources and definitions. Journal of Marriage and Family 62(3): 655

Whitley E, Gunnell D, Dorling D et al 1999 Ecological study of social fragmentation, poverty and suicide. British Medical Journal 319: 1034–1037

World Health Organisation 1992 The ICD-10 classification of mental and behavioural disorders: clinical description and diagnostic guidelines. WHO, Geneva

World Health Organisation 2000 WHO issues new healthy life expectancy rankings. Press release, Washington DC and Geneva, 4 June 2000. Online. Available: http://www.who.int/inf-pr-2000/en/pr2000-life.html

Further reading

Department of Health 2000 National service framework for coronary heart disease. Department of Health, London

Forrester DA 1996 Myths of masculinity: impact upon men's health. Nursing Clinics of North America 21(1): 19

Lane SD, Cibula DA 2000 Gender and Health. In: Albrecht GL, Fitzpatrick R (eds) The handbook of social studies in health and medicine. Sage, London

Petersen S, Rayner M 2002 Coronary heart disease statistics. British Heart Foundation statistics database. British Heart Foundation, London, p. 1–164

Ruxton S 2001 Men, masculinities and poverty. Oxfam, Oxford

Ziguras C 1998 Masculinity and self care. In: Laws T (ed) Promoting men's health: an essential book for nurses. Ausmed, Australia

Resources

Aldridge D 2000 Spirituality, healing and medicine: return to the silence. Jessica Kingsley, London

American Psychiatric Association 2000 Diagnostic and statistical manual of mental disorder, 4th edn. (DSM IV) APA, Washington DC

DOH 2003 National partnership agreement on the transfer of responsibility for prison health from the Home Office to the Department of Health. Online. Available: http://www.doh.gov.uk/prisonhealth/npafinal.PDF

HMPS 2003 Prison health handbook. Prison Health Policy Unit and Task Force. Online. Available: http://www.hmprisonservice.gov.uk/filestore/1033_1428.pdf

ICD-9-CM International Classification of Diseases. Mental disorders can be located in classification number 290–319. Online. Available: http://www.newcastle.edu.au/centre/hsrg/hypertexts/icd9cm.html

Koenig HG 2000 Religion, spirituality and medicine: application to clinical practice. JAMA 284(13): 1708

Mental health policy implementation guide 2001. Online. Available: http://www.doh.gov.uk/mentalhealth/implementationguide.htm

Reforming the Mental Health Act. Department of Health. Online. Available: http://www.doh.gov.uk/mentalhealth/whitepaper2000.htm

Ronaldson S (ed) 1997 Spirituality: the heart of nursing. Ausmed Publication, Melbourne

US Department of Health and Human Services, National Institutes of Health, National Institutes of Mental Health. National Institute of Mental Health – Real men, real depression http://menanddepression.nimh.nih.gov/ This web site can be used for clients who would like to know more about their depression. It details symptoms and treatments for depression, gives personal stories and publications, fact sheets.

Chapter 2

Promoting health

CHAPTER CONTENTS

HEALTH PROMOTION

Defining health promotion

The education of individuals and groups about health and prevention of illness has been described as 'health promotion'. However, this definition has broadened rapidly since the 1970s and now encompasses the health of populations and communities in a global context. The term health promotion is now difficult to separate from terms such as 'primary health care', 'public health', 'new public health' and 'community health' because the boundaries between them are not constant and there may be overlapping meanings to each (Baum, 2002 p. 530).

Policy development in health promotion

The *Ottawa Charter for Health Promotion* (WHO 1986) was the primary outcome from the first WHO International Conference on Health Promotion held in Ottawa, Canada, in 1986. The Ottawa Charter sets out lines of action required to achieve the declaration 'Health for all by the year 2000'. Health promotion 'lines of action' refers to the building of healthy public policy, creating supportive environments, strengthening community action, developing personal skills, and reorientating health services. **Men's health policy** development, limited as it is, focuses on these aspects of the charter (see section on policy development in the *Preface*).

Underpinning the call for **social justice** are the principles of:

- equitable access to resources that promote health
- community participation
- socially acceptable and affordable technology
- the provision of health services based on the needs of the population
- health education and work to improve the root cause of ill health. (Declaration of Alma-Ata, WHO 1978, http://www.who.int/hpr/NPH/docs/declaration_almaata.pdf)

Importantly, the tenet of *gender equity* has now been linked to other factors influencing health status (i.e. equitable access to appropriate health care and resources as explained in Chapter 1).

Enabling health promotion

The WHO identifies broader social elements that 'enable' health promotion to occur; they are: 'Any combination of health education and related organisational, political and economic intervention designed to facilitate behavioural and environmental adaptations which will improve health.' (Anderson 1983).

Helping men change

For there to be a sustainable change in the provision of health services for men and boys, with the aim of improving the health status, there is a necessary requirement of developing valid and reliable data on men's perception of health, their health practices and their health needs. It is also fundamental that health researchers incorporate into their research methods (examples of methods include interviews and questionnaires) some questions about gender, and develop methodologies (the way the data are viewed and interpreted) that increasingly focus on the nexus between masculinity and health practices. Gender is an important item for researchers to consider because women also influence what is expected of men vis-à-vis their health knowledge and practices.

Key points

- Men should not be considered as a homogenous group by policy makers and service providers.
- Health promotion activities need to be designed for men rather than on a population base or as an adjunct to women's health promotion activities.
- Policy makers and practitioners will need to develop an understanding of the nexus between gender and health when formulating specific interventions/services for men.
- All health policies should incorporate gender as a theme when evaluating the needs of a group at risk.

Health promoting activities

It is because nurses have first hand experience of men's health issues that they can and do play an important role in developing and conducting promotion activities. Here are some examples:

- Community screening programmes (glaucoma, hypertension, diabetes)
- Annual health assessments relative to age, risk and sex (GPs)
- Being proactive in seeking help from health professionals
- Lifestyle rehabilitation programmes (alcohol, gambling, smoking)
- Stress management programmes (work, marriage, divorce)
- Money and debt advisors (see section below on Health issues nominated by men)
- Sexual and reproductive health services
- Self care programmes/maintaining social activities and contact
- Knowledge sharing within and among communities
- Working with local schools (school canteens, prevention of bullying)

- Joining and supporting national health and consumer groups, (e.g. Action on Smoking and Health (ASH))
- Accessing websites (e.g. The Health Protection Agency, UK http://www.hpa.org.uk/default.htm)
- The UK's first national men's health week was held in June 2002.

Nurses also need to show to policy makers and those that fund health care that nurse led health promotion activities do make a difference. This requires that nurses become more involved in publicising evaluations of the programmes and men's health activities; too often this stage is not planned for or followed through.

What are men's health promotion resources?

- The GP was nominated by 42% of people as their healthier lifestyle advisor.
- Health promotion messages/leaflets from GP's waiting rooms and community health services.
- Twice as many men as women, aged 30–59, chose a family member as a healthier lifestyle advisor
- Internet coverage of men's health issues is improving. However, the layman has difficulty identifying gaps and inaccuracies in this literature and all too often the information is linked to product marking (Berland 2001).

Printed material and advertising are not a panacea

Overall, everyday practice evidence based leaflets have not been effective in promoting informed choice (Wicke et al 1994):

- Health promotion messages/leaflets are read by less than 10% of patients in UK GP's waiting rooms.
- Some health professionals have withheld leaflets on the basis that many either suggested choices that were not available locally or were at odds with staff beliefs.
- Health promotional messages emanating from electronic notice boards and videos in GP's waiting rooms may detract from the waiting rooms other functions (e.g. patients mentally preparing their case history on current episode of illness).

Despite these negative reports health professionals should, as a point of best practice and for medicolegal reasons, provide patients with information leaflets as they are an efficient means of reiterating salient points made during consultation.

HEALTH ISSUES NOMINATED BY MEN

What do men believe are the issues?

The vast majority of men's health issues have been generated out of epidemiological studies showing that men have higher rates of mortality and morbidity than women. However, few researchers have asked men what issues they hold. A study by Fletcher & Higginbotham (2001) offers rare insights into what men believe are the main health issues. Of the 312 Australian men responding to open ended questions, 84% chose the following as the main items for concern:

- Alcohol
- Smoking
- Heart disease
- Overweight.

The top 10 health concerns (from a list of 52 items) were:

- Stress
- Skin cancer
- Tiredness
- Back problems*
- Heart disease
- Road traffic accident
- Lack of exercise
- Disturbed sleep
- Money problems
- Overweight.

* Back problems were experienced by 40% of men compared to 12% in an earlier National Health Survey.

These men would have liked more help for dealing with their:

- Stress and the cost of medical care
- Money problems
- Back problems
- Job satisfaction
- Dissatisfaction with quality of medical care
- Tiredness
- Disturbed sleep

- Lack of exercise
- Poor access to medical care.

The responses to Fletcher and Higginbotham's survey are mainly concerned with men's ability to fulfil their role as breadwinner. For unemployed men, their health concerns, experiences and priorities were clearly dominated by employment status. The responses strongly suggest that most men have substantial unmet health needs (Fletcher & Higginbotham 2001). Arguably, nurses should, where possible, incorporate these items as questions into a holistic health assessment of the adult male patient.

Young males

Only 5% of total deaths occur among young adults, yet a third of these are attributable to injury, poisoning and accidents and are therefore considered 'avoidable'. Alcohol-related mortality has risen in young adult males and females, to the extent that it has almost tripled between 1979 and 2001. Deaths from drug-related poisoning have tripled among the young between 1979 and 2001 to a rate of 13% in young males and 7% in young females (Brock & Griffiths 2003). (See Chapter 4 'Young men' for detailed sections on 'alcohol abuse' and 'substance abuse'). From the 1990s suicide has become more common among young males (see Chapter 1, the section on suicide).

Obesity and overweight males

Assessing obesity and weight (adults)

Two indicators are used by nurses and GPs to determine the need for weight loss: the body mass index (BMI) and measurement of total body fatness.

The distribution of body fat is also an important factor in assessing the risk of myocardial infarction. The higher the distribution of upper body fat, the greater the risk of health problems. Strategies for losing weight should be actively pursued for men with high levels of upper body fat even though health problems are not evident.

Body mass index

A BMI is calculated by dividing weight in kilograms by height in metres squared. BMI levels in adults are customarily grouped into grades (see Table 2.1). A BMI between 25 and 30 is considered as overweight and > 30 dictates a weight loss programme be commenced for treatment of obesity (< 18.5 suggests the man is underweight). However, there is no similar agreed grouping in children.

UK data

Obesity is a health problem for many younger men. Within the age group of 16–24 years 23% (male) and 19% (female) were identified as overweight and 6% (male) and 8% (female) were classified obese. There were no clear relationships between male BMI and social class or household income.

Australian data

Australia is ranked as one of the fattest developed nations, closely following USA. Data shows that the rate of the 'overweight' and 'obese' adult (> 25 years) has almost doubled amongst Australians over the last two decades.

- Overweight men 67% and women 53%
- Obesity in females 22% compared to men 19% (AIHW 2003a)

Health implications of abnormal weight gain

- Hypertension
- Hyperlipidaemia
- Increased insulin resistance and glucose intolerance
- Increased risk of diabetes
- Increased risk of coronary heart disease
- Social ostracism.

Table 2.1   BMI grades

BMI grades	Classification
20 kg/m² or less	underweight
20–25 kg/m²	desirable weight
25–30 kg/m²	overweight
over 30 kg/m²	obese

Benefits of losing weight

Data from the Framingham study (Harris et al 1988) showed that a 10% reduction in body weight among overweight men resulted on average in :

- a fall in serum glucose of 2.5 mg/dL
- a fall in serum cholesterol of 11.3 mg/dL
- a fall in systolic blood pressure of 6.6 mmHg
- a fall in uric acid of 0.33 mg/dL.

Nurses assisting men in weight loss programmes or nutritional health promotional activities should emphasise that it is not necessary to achieve ideal body weight in order to reap health benefits. Most health benefits are gained with modest weight loss. For example, for every 10% reduction in weight there is a concomitant reduction in the risk of coronary heart disease of 20%.

Accident and illness prevention

Over the last four decades mortality rates have decreased for both men and women, the exception to this has been for those aged 15–44 years. Although mortality from 'land transport accidents' and most diseases decreased for young adults this has been offset by increases in deaths from suicide, alcohol and drug poisoning. These health problems are considered preventable and consequently considerable research is being undertaken to develop health promotion strategies in these areas (Brock & Griffiths 2003). The UK government has responded by developing several strategies to prevent these problems and has set health targets to be met.

Some health strategies introduced by the UK Department of Health

- National suicide prevention strategy for England (DH, NIMME 2005)
- Government response to the advisory council on the Misuse of Drugs Report into drug related deaths (Department of Health 2001)
- National alcohol harm reduction strategy (Department of Health 2002).

Health targets

These include:

* death rates from accidents and suicide to be reduced by 20% (2010)
* death by road accidents by 40% (2010).

Has anything worked for young men so far (UK)?

Even though **road accidents** have historically caused greater mortality and morbidity among young males than females, recent figures show improvements have taken place. Although the number of licensed motor vehicles increased by 68% in the UK for the period 1976–2001, the mortality rates for men declined. This has been attributed to the compulsory wearing of seatbelts (introduced in 1965 and for back seat passengers in 1991) and the introduction of the alcohol breathalyser test (1976).

For young adult men, the mortality rates attributable to **IHD, stroke and lung cancer** fell between the mid 1970s and 2000. This trend followed that seen in men at older ages (Brock & Griffiths 2003).

Brock and Griffiths (2003) examined the causes of death for young adults and found that over the past four decades:

* all causes of mortality for adults (defined as >15 years) decreased
* the age-standardised mortality rate for all causes of death fell 40% for males and females.

However, death rates ceased to decline for young men from the late 1980s and mortality rates for young men levelled off in the early 1990s. This phenomenon has been attributed in part to alcohol-related deaths, HIV/AIDS deaths and drug-related mortalities. From baseline data from the 1980s to 2001 there has been a 7% increase in alcohol-related mortalities in young adult men. The main cause of death in older adult males is cirrhosis of the liver. Alcohol-related deaths for men aged 15–44 years were higher than those in women and the trend line has been much steeper for men since the early 1990s. Drug-related mortalities were higher for men from the 1990s and have peaked at three times the rate of women. Drug-related poisonings have tripled for young men between 1979 and 2001. HIV/AIDS accounted for only 3% of all male deaths in young adults in 1995.

Alcohol

The term alcohol refers generally to multiple organic compounds, of which only ethyl alcohol or ethanol can be consumed with relative safety by humans. Patterns of alcohol misuse vary according to time in history, age, sex and ethnicity (Simpura & Karlsson 2001). Approximately 10% of adults consume alcohol at risky levels. The prevalence of alcohol dependence in Australia, according to the DSM–VI specificaton is estimated to be 4.1% with abuse at 1.9% (Degenhardt et al 2000). In the UK 39% of men and 23% of women in 2000 had drunk in excess of the daily recommended levels (HAD 2002). The relationship between increasing alcohol consumption and increasing risk of harm/poorer health is robust. Social factors include higher risk of relationship breakdown, criminal violence (victim or perpetrator), road traffic and work place accidents and suicide. Common health-related problems include oesophageal varices, oesophageal cancer, cirrhosis of the liver, pancreatitis and dementia.

Measuring intake

A standard drink of alcohol is 10 grams (12.5 millilitres of ethanol). However, since drinks come in different size glasses it may be challenging to calculate consumption in scientific terms (standard drinks/grams of alcohol). Consequently, there is a stong argument for calculating consumption on the basis of a 'standard unit'. The standard unit is the measure used in the United Kingdom (NHMRC 2001).

How much do men drink?

In England in 2001, almost 38% of men had drunk 4 units of alcohol or more on at least one day in the previous week and 22% of women had drunk 3 units or more over the same period. In 2001, 27% of men and 15% of women aged 16 and over drank, on average, more than 21 and 14 units a week respectively. Drinking at these levels among men has remained stable at about 27% since 1992 (Department of Health 2003).

What are the health effects of alcohol?

Road traffic accidents: estimates from data for 2002 showed that 6% of road traffic accidents involved illegal blood alcohol levels, and that these accidents resulted in a total of 20 140 casualties (Department of Health 2003).

Alcohol-related deaths: in the early 1980s, in the UK, 2% of deaths among young adults were alcohol-related. This has risen by 7% for young males and 6% for young females. However, in the older age group, mortality rates in men were higher than those of women. There was a steep increase in alcohol related deaths in men and women aged 35–44 from the mid 1980s with rates doubling in both sexes in the 40–44 age group during that time (Brock & Griffiths 2003). In Australia approximately 70% of the 3290 alcohol-related deaths recorded in 1997 were male deaths (NHMRC 2001). These figures indicate a substantial health problem in many countries.

The World Health Organisation (WHO) Working Group on alcohol and health identified two different approaches to the reduction of alcohol misuse and alcohol-related harm (WHO Working Group 1995).

- to persuade individuals to drink in a certain way by the provision of information and advice
- to change the drinker's environment to help shape drinking patterns and drinking contexts (Health Development Agency 2002).

Level of risk for men

- The consumption of 3–4 standard drinks per day holds no more risk of premature death relative to non-drinkers.
- The consumption of 6 or more standard drinks per day is associated with significant risk in the short term.
- There is limited evidence to suggest that 1–2 standard drinks per day may have cardiac benefits for men aged over 45 (drink is not necessary to achieve these gains; exercise, stopping smoking and following a balanced diet are preferable).

Alcohol-related problems

- 6% of alcohol related deaths were caused by alcoholic liver cirrhosis, road accidents, stroke, suicide and alcohol dependence.
- Other health concerns include alcohol-related violence, alcohol-related assault.
- 65% of alcohol related hospitalisations in 1996–1997 were attributed to injuries sustained from falls, assaults and road accidents.

- Men drinking at high-risk levels will find it difficult to achieve an erection and long term effects will result in impotence.
- Heavy drinking is a high-risk behaviour for suicidal ideation/self-harm and suicide (NHMRC 2001).

Guidelines for minimising risk

Minimise intoxication (short term problem) by drinking a maximum of 2 standard drinks in the first hour and then no more than one drink per hour thereafter. To minimise long term problems men should follow these guidelines:

- Drink no more than 6 standard drinks per day.
- Drink *on average* no more than 4 standard drinks per day.
- Drink no more than 28 standard drinks per week.
- Don't drink on 2 days of the week.
- The levels set in these guidelines may be too high for men with lower BMI (N.B. 17% of men and women are underweight in the UK).

These guidelines assume that the drinker is not on medication, does not have a family history of alcohol-related problems or a medical condition made worse by the consumption of alcohol.

How do nurses detect an alcohol problem? (New South Wales Department of Health 2000, NDARC 2003)

People who abuse alcohol often hide the extent to which they consume it. Therefore it takes a skilled clinician to detect the problem and raise the proposition of creating an effective plan to assist clients to reduce consumption or stop their intake altogether.

As a *preliminary step* to detecting a problem the nurse can and should use:

- linking reason for admission to medical service with alcohol
- general interview data/client history, with a direct question about consumption rate and amount
- assessment for visible physical signs (see a nursing textbook).

Common physical manifestations of alcohol abuse are:

- Dilated facial capillaries
- Bloodshot eyes
- Fine tremor of hand or tongue.

Diagnosis

Effective diagnosis requires the use of a variety of techniques for gathering information about the person. Effective diagnostic assessment commonly includes the use of :

● Diagnostic interviews used with a screening tool (questionnaire).
● Standardised and validated questionnaires
● Nursing examination of client
● Data from medical examination (enlarged liver, hypertension)
● Biological markers.

N. B. Details of these diagnostic items and their effectiveness are provided in specific upcoming sections.

Medical history

● Gastrointestinal disorders
● Duodenal ulcers
● Acute pancreatitis
● Use of medications

Biological markers: are they effective in diagnosis?

A wide range of markers offers the opportunity to provide the client with evidence of a physiological problem. Men seem to be particularly partial to empirical evidence as a means of persuasion towards modifying their risk factors. Such markers include:

● Serum GGT
● Aspartate (AST)
● Alanine amino transferase (ALT)
● HDL – cholesterol
● Uric acid
● Mean cell volume (elevated MCV is found in < 20% of alcoholics)
● Carbohydrate-deficient transferrin (CDT). Test kits are available in some clinics.

Many of these biological changes are reversible because of the liver's capacity to compensate for diminution of hepatocytes.

Whilst a combination of markers can improve the chance of detecting an alcohol problem (sensitivity of 78% – i.e. few false positives) such combinations are not recommended for clinical practice because of a reduced level of specificity (greater chance of false negatives). A questionnaire approach to detecting alcohol problems is preferred to a reliance on only biological markers because these tools, such as the alcohol use disorder identification test (AUDIT) questionnaire, have greater sensitivity and specificity.

N. B. The AUDIT tool is described in a later section.

Are screening tools effective?

There is strong evidence to show that health professionals within hospitals and general practice can effectively screen for and intervene to off-set risky alcohol consumption. The AUDIT and quantity frequency index (retrospective diary) are recommended for use in the hospital setting, general practice, community health care and the workplace (NDRAC 2003).

Clinical interviews for alcohol abuse

A greater richness of data will come from the nurse's use of open-ended questioning and the avoidance of questioning by checklist as the latter often constrains the type and length of responses men and women make.

Items to be explored in the psychosocial interview include but are not limited to:

- Family discord
- Work place tension/unemployment
- History of violence/assault/injury (previous hospital admission)
- History of sexual abuse
- Military service and PTSD.

Specific items to be explored in the mental state interview include:

- Anxieties
- Physical status/wellness (signs of tremulousness, hyper-reflexia, insomnia)
- Depression
- Cognitive impairment
- Psychosis.

Probing questions that can be used to explore drinking/drug use include:

- What time do you start drinking?
- Do you ever drink in the morning?
- Tell me what you drank over the week (leaving out nothing)?
- Have you ever felt you should cut down?
- Have people annoyed you by criticising your drinking?
- Have you ever felt guilty about your drinking?

Key points (NDARC 2003)

A semi-structured interview, where there is guided exploration of the client's subjective experience of his drinking, is far better than a vague, directionless discussion of the drinker's general history.

Interviewers should cover the following areas:

- Presenting problem
- Role of drinking in presenting problem
- Identification of the reason/motivation for change
- Adjunct concerns (work, family, legal, financial problems).

Including family members in the assessment phase can provide valuable information concerning alcohol-related problems at home and in the workplace, along with what triggers drinking and what typifies his drinking pattern.

Information about past experiences is important. Past experiences are helpful in clarifying how the man came to be in the present situation and what is maintaining maladaptive thoughts and behaviours.

The interviewer should be cognisant of the likelihood of alcohol related brain damage and be observing for signs of neuropathology during the interview (*see section on assessing memory and cognitive function below*).

Assessment should lead to an agreed set of treatment goals and the formalisation of a treatment plan.

Assessing memory and cognitive function

The NDARC (2003) states that if a man over the age of 45 has been drinking to excess for 15 years or more and reports some social and/or vocational disruption, this indicates that some form of alcohol-related brain damage or reduction of cognitive function has taken place. Clients with this profile are likely to relate problems associated with planning activities and problem solving to health professionals interviewing them. Cognitive impairment may extend to impairment of verbal communication, visual and spatial abilities.

Profound short term memory loss occurs with Wernicke Korsakoff's syndrome (WKS) with only some long term recall of events remaining intact. Lack of retention of new information has wide implications for clients' educational needs. These men cannot rely on memory alone to make changes to drinking and nutritional habits. However, substantial improvement in cognition can be gained, within a short period, from the daily use of thiamine (vitamin B1) supplements in combination with a continuation of abstinence. An intramuscular injection of 100 mg of thiamine per day can be prescribed for 3 days. If this route is contraindicated then oral administration (100 mg of thiamine, three times per day, for at least a week) can be used.

If the nurse suspects that a person has cognitive impairment, as evidenced by a **mini mental health assessment** (see Box 2.1), then a referral to a doctor and subsequent referral to a psychologist or neuropsychologist is appropriate.

Are questionnaires equally effective for men as women?

The AUDIT questionnaire is equally effective for both sexes and across cultural groups. The AUDIT is also effective irrespective of whether it is used as an interview questionnaire or a self-administered questionnaire. Women are somewhat disadvantaged in getting to centres to be assessed as many health centres do not have childcare facilities. This problem is compounded because many women with alcohol problems perceive that females are stereotyped as not being able to care for their families. Consequently, these women hold a fear of losing their children.

Mental health problems commonly coexist with alcohol misuse and many homeless men are homeless as a consequence of mental health problems. This co-morbidity means it is difficult to reach these men for assessment and treatment. The T-ACE and TWEAK instruments shown in Boxes 2.2 and 2.3 have better specificity and sensitivity with respect to detecting problem drinking among pregnant women, relative to MAST or CAGE. (MAST is a self-

Box 2.1   Assessing cognitive function (Baldwin 1979)

The primary function of a 'mini mental health assessment' is to measure cognitive function. The tests take approximately 10 minutes to administer when used by a practised clinician, and include:

- Orientation in the following chronology (year, season, date, day, month)
- Orientation in place (state, country, hospital, level/floor)
- Registration (naming three objects, individually then collectively)
- Attention and calculation (counting backwards from 100 in units of 7)
- Attention and calculation (spelling the word 'world' backwards)
- Recall (repeating the three objects cited earlier in the test)
- Language

naming objects, repeating phrases
obeying commands that incorporate three steps
writing a sentence
copying a design

Where difficulty in reading and/or writing is detected the nurse will need to adjust the tool (e.g. use large print text for those with visual impairment).

Box 2.2   Screening instrument T–ACE

This is quick and easy to administer and a score of > 2 indicates clients may be drinking to a level that is damaging their health and further assessment is needed to verify that risk level.

T = **Tolerance**: how many drinks are needed for you to feel the effects

A = Are you **annoyed** by people who question/criticise your drinking?

C = Have you *ever* felt that you needed to **cut down** your drinking?

E = Have you ever had a drink soon after waking, an **eye opener**, to steady your disposition/nerves?

Box 2.3   Screening instrument TWEAK

A score of > 2 is indicative of the client consuming alcohol to risky levels.

T =   **Tolerance:** how many drinks are you able to hold?

W =   Have close friends or family been **worried** or complained about your drinking over the past year?

E =   **Eye opener:** are there times when you drink soon after getting up?

A =   **Amnesia:** have close friends or family told you things that you have not remembered?

K (C) = do you have **knowledge** of wanting to **cut down?**

administered questionnaire of 24 items designed to identify a physiological dependence on alcohol and alcohol abuse; CAGE is a 4 item screening tool designed to identify a physiological dependence on alcohol and alcohol abuse. It is less sensitive than AUDIT or the MAST tool because of the brief data collected.)

AUDIT screening instrument

The alcohol use disorder identification test screening instrument (AUDIT) was developed and evaluated for over 2 decades and has been found to provide an accurate means of measuring risk across gender, age and cultures. The AUDIT is recommended for screening psychiatric populations (NDARC 2003).

As the first screening test to be designed for use specifically in a primary health care setting the AUDIT has the following advantages:

- Cross-national standardisation: the AUDIT was validated on primary health care patients in six countries. It is the only screening test specifically designed for international use.
- Identifies hazardous and harmful alcohol use, as well as possible dependence.
- Brief, rapid and flexible.
- Designed for use by primary healthcare workers.
- Consistent with ICD–10 definitions of alcohol dependence and harmful alcohol use.

- Focuses on recent alcohol use. (*WHO website*
  http://www.who.int/substanceabuse/activities/sbi/en/)

The AUDIT questionnaire is too large to include in this hand-book. However, you can download it in the AUDIT manual from the WHO web address above or directly using: http://whqlibdoc. who.int/hq/2001/WHO_MSD_MSB_01.6a.pdf

Withdrawal from alcohol

Experience suggests that levels of consumption do not predict the severity of the withdrawal. Individuals can react very differently to cessation of alcohol irrespective of the pattern and level of drinking. No nurses want their patients, who have been admitted for conditions other than alcohol abuse, to surprise them by exhibiting signs of alcohol withdrawal. Given the widespread use and abuse of alcohol it is prudent to assess all patients for alcohol use as a means of identifying the probability of withdrawal.

Withdrawal rating scale

The person with a past history of withdrawal symptoms or seizure should be monitored carefully using a withdrawal rating scale and regime that stipulates a maximum time between nursing observations (see CIWA_AR withdrawal scale a copy of which can be obtained from the Clinical Institute Withdrawal Assessment for Alcohol website: http://www.fpnotebook.com/PSY75.htm

Symptom onset

Those physically dependent on alcohol are likely to experience withdrawal symptoms 6–24 hours after their last drink was consumed.

Seizures

Withdrawal seizures can occur from 12–48 hours after the last drink consumed.

Delirium tremens (DTs)

These are a serious complication of withdrawal, occurring 48–96 hours after cessation and can be life-threatening. Hypotension, dehydration, renal failure and pneumonia are ominous signs. Sedation, intravenous fluid replacement and sedations are essential treatments.

Signs of withdrawal (not in order of occurence)

- Hyperthermia
- Tachycardia
- Tachypnoea
- Hypertension
- Nausea and vomiting
- Tremor
- Diaphoresis
- Agitation, hyperactivity
- Sleep disturbance
- Tactile disturbance (pins and needles, burning, itching, something crawling over skin)
- Auditory and visual hallucinations
- Perceptual distortions
- Anxiety
- Paranoid delusions
- Abnormal affect (see above for mental health assessment and explanation).

Drug management

Diazepam is considered the first line of treatment and gold standard for the management of alcohol withdrawal. Diazepam, an anti-anxiety agent, can be prescribed as 20 mg every 2 hours until the withdrawal subsides. However, there are alternative regimes for the drug that run over 2–6 days.

Key points

Symptoms of withdrawal can become apparent before the person's blood alcohol level (BAL) reaches zero and so observations for withdrawal should begin even when the BAL is well above zero.

A patient withdrawing from alcohol may be withdrawing from other drugs or reacting to other drugs taken after alcohol was ceased.

Although withdrawal symptoms are self limiting and are usually resolved within 5 days, some individuals have an increasing severity of symptoms throughout the period of 48–72 hours of abstinence, and seizures can occur between 12 and 48 hours after cessation.

Key points—cont'd

Alcohol withdrawal rating scales are designed to detect and monitor the severity of the withdrawal but should not be used as a diagnostic tool (NDARC 2003).

Home-based withdrawal

Some people have their withdrawal managed within their own home or group accommodation setting. This can be arranged provided there is supportive care and a reliable telephone referral service accessible over 24 hours and 7 days per week. Suitable individuals are those with no significant medical or psychiatric history, no past history of severe withdrawal symptoms and/or heavy use of alcohol over prolonged periods. For those men who have a partner with an alcohol problem the home-based withdrawal service offers many benefits. Their spouse/partner can be in a non-threatening environment and the need to find child care for a hospitalisation or clinic admission could not be used as a reason for not attempting a planned withdrawal.

Referrals to special services

Spend some time noting the telephone help lines for people with drug and alcohol problems in your country and identify local agencies and recommended resources to assist those that are seeking help. You can use a grid such as that shown in Figure 2.1.

Smoking

Do male and female smoking rates differ?

Although rates of smoking among men have reduced substantially over the last two decades in many countries rates remain above

RESOURCE	Agency	Address	Web site	Ph number
Help line				
Resources				
Counselling service				

Figure 2.1   Grid for recording support services and agencies.

those of women. Tables 2.2 and 2.3 show figures for Australia and the UK.

Is smoking more hazardous for males?

The total number of deaths attributed to smoking in the UK in 1997 was 75 600 for males and 43 200 for females (total = 118 800). Treating diseases caused by smoking costs the NHS in the region of £1.5 billion a year. People who smoke and drink alcohol regularly are at greater risk of mouth and throat cancers. Men have higher rates of combining alcohol and tobacco smoking and the effects of this are evident in Table 2.4.

Does smoking affect male reproduction?

Smoking increases the risk of erectile dysfunction by around 50% for men in their 30s and 40s. Smoking can also interfere with fertility by:

• Reducing the volume of ejaculate
• Lowering sperm count
• Contributing to abnormal sperm shape
• Impairing sperm motility (ASH 2004, BMA 2004).

Can nurses help men quit smoking?

Nurses are in a position to advise men on the links between ill health/diseases and cancer. If men are receptive to this message

Table 2.2 Percentage of Australian adults who smoke (QUIT 2005)

Year	1954	1964	1969	1974	1976	1980	1983	1986	1989	1992	1995
Male	72	58	45	45	43	41	40	33	30	28	27
Female	26	28	28	30	30	31	31	29	27	24	23

Table 2.3 Percentage of UK adults who smoke (ASH 2005)

Year	1974	1978	1982	1986	1990	1994	1996	1998	2000	2001
Male	51	45	38	35	31	28	29	28	29	28
Female	41	37	33	31	29	26	28	26	25	26

Table 2.4 Smoking statistics related to illness types (QUIT 2005)

	Number of men	Number of women	Total	% of all deaths from disease (men)	% of all deaths from disease (women)
Cancer					
Lung	19 600	9 600	29 200	89	75
Upper respiratory	1500	400	1900	74	50
Oesophagus	2900	1700	4600	71	65
Bladder	1600	300	1900	47	19
Kidney	700	100	800	40	6
Stomach	1600	300	1900	35	11
Pancreas	600	900	1500	20	26
Unspecified site	2400	600	3000	33	7
Myeloid leukaemia	200	100	300	19	11
Respiratory					
Chronic obstructive lung disease	14 000	9700	23 700	86	81
Pneumonia	5600	4800	10 500	23	13
Circulatory					
Ischaemic heart disease	16 800	7500	24 300		

and declare that they would like to stop smoking, then nurses should provide men with a fact sheet on how to stop, using the ASH website http://www.ash.org.uk/. The basic points are:

- Get professional help
- Prepare mentally
- Dispel smoking myths
- Know what to expect
- Make a list of reasons why you want to stop
- Consider the money spent

- Set a date
- Involve friends and family
- Deal with nicotine withdrawal
- Other treatments may help
- Find a (temporary) substitute habit
- Deal with any weight-gain worries
- Avoid temptation
- Stop completely
- Watch out for relapse.

SCREENING

The concept

The concept of screening is based on the assumption that disease is preceded by a period of asymptomatic pathogenesis (disease development). Screening techniques seek to identify this otherwise hidden pathogenesis. Screening is not considered to be a diagnostic test; it simply raises sufficient suspicion for the physician to order diagnostic tests on a seemingly healthy individual.

A definition

'The systematic application of a test or inquiry, to identify individuals at sufficient risk of a specific disorder to warrant further investigations or direct preventive action, amongst persons who have not sought medical attention on account of symptoms of that disorder.' (NSC 1998, p. 12)

Objectives of a screening test

1. **A high sensitivity is desirable** (i.e. few *false negatives*): a low sensitivity means there is a high risk of a false negative. In this case the patient may be told the results are negative but they actually have the disease.
2. **A high specificity is desirable** (i.e. few *false positives*): a low specificity means there is a high risk of a false positive. A patient may be told that the results are positive but the result is not conclusive. Consequently, further tests are needed to determine whether or not there is a false positive. These additional tests may have harmful side effects or complications.
3. **The benefits should outweigh the harm** to the individual that arises as a consequence of screening.

4. **A high positive predictive value** (PPV) is desirable: the equation for PPV reflects the specificity and sensitivity as well as the prevalence of the disease in the population.

Developing a screening programme

Screening programmes should be based on a set of agreed principles rather than be developed on the basis of an *ad hoc* process designed to address anxieties held by individuals or communities (see 'Debates on screening').

Screening programmes should be based upon the following principles:

- The condition should pose an important health problem.
- There should be a recognisable early stage of the disease (evidence of pathological changes).
- Early treatment should be proven to be more beneficial than later treatment.
- A test should be found that has a high PPV.
- At risk populations and subgroups of the population should be defined as at risk.
- At risk populations should have priority for screening.
- A rationale for the recommended frequency of screening needs to be developed.
- An assessment needs to be made of the costs and benefits to the individual and healthcare body. (Austoker 1995)

Debates on screening

The media and health promotional agencies have successfully conveyed the message to the public that screening saves lives because earlier detection of a disease means earlier treatment. However, the medical profession is considering whether some screening methods are ethical and effective in terms of improving patient outcomes. (Raffle et al (2003) estimate that for cervical cancer 1000 women have to be screened for 35 years to prevent one death, and Tang et al (2004) preposed that the extent to which GPs support population-based colorectal screening remains unclear.) Currently under debate is screening for prostate cancer and testicular cancer. GPs have been informed by specialist medical groups that it is entirely inappropriate to screen for prostate cancer, and may even be harmful. Yet many GPs continue to screen and men requesting screening do not understand the issues involved (Laws et al 2000).

Screening guidelines for prostate cancer

The guidelines stating that screening for prostate cancer should not be done are supported by the knowledge that current tests, i.e. prostate specific antigen (PSA), digital rectal examination (DRE) and transrectal ultrasound, are not accurate. Moreover, none of these tests or combinations of tests have been linked to a means of reducing mortality from this cancer. Further, a test with a positive result may be a false positive and it may require a per-rectal biopsy of the prostate to confirm this. However, the procedure is not without risk of haemorrhage, septicaemia and psychological stress (Taylor 1993, Hirst 1996). Despite guidelines, men continue to request screening and GPs continue to use these tests to screen. The rationale for this lies in GPs' fear of litigation, what if they refuse to provide the tests and the man later develop prostate cancer.

Why are tests for prostate cancer unreliable?

- DRE has limited sensitivity. 'DRE is limited in that only the posterior and lateral aspects of the prostate can be palpated, thus 40–50 per cent of cancers are beyond reach.' (Sladden 1993, p. 1386).
- A large number of serum PSA results are false positive results (low specificity), precluding it as a single screening tool (Hirst 1996). Proving a false positive requires a biopsy of the prostate.
- The PSA test has a low sensitivity (higher than acceptable risk of false negative). For example, Punglia et al (2003) found that from 6691 screened, 82% of men in the under 60 years group had a *normal PSA level* even though *they had prostate cancer* confirmed. This indicates that the PSA test has a low sensitivity, a high risk of a false negative. The danger is that patients may be told the results are negative but they actually have the disease.
- Only a few studies have shown that by using a ratio of free-to-total PSA the specificity of the test is raised significantly.
- Although transrectal ultrasound has a low sensitivity when used alone and even when used in conjunction with information, the detection rate for a lesion that is localised may be low (Austoker 1995).

Testicular cancer screening is not widespread

Testicular self examination (TSE) is a common method of screening for testicular cancer (TC). Arguments against screening rest on lack of evidence to show that it is effective or necessary because:

- Testicular tumours are uncommon (1% of all cancers in males).
- There is no conclusive evidence to show that men with TC identified through screening have better health outcomes from treatment than those men who present with clinical signs later in the disease.
- The cure rate is rising (95–100%) despite the current poor uptake of TSE.
- It is argued that funds spent on screening could be better spent elsewhere. For example, 1 in 12 men will have lung cancer.

Testicular self examination (TSE)

Figures 2.2a and 2.2b below indicate the two simple steps to this procedure which can easily be performed monthly whilst showering. It is important to know the normal geography of the scrotum and its contents. For example, a difference in the size of the testes is normal for many men and one may hang lower than the other. The surface of the testis should feel firm and smooth.

- **Step one:** Roll a testicle gently between thumb and forefinger, then progress to the other. Feel for lumps the size of a pea in or on the surface of the testis, or a change to the contour. Lumps are generally painless.
- **Step two:** Using thumb and forefinger, feel along the back of the testis. The epididymis, the tube carrying sperm from the testis, should be soft and non-tender.

Symptoms suggestive of a growth also include:

- A feeling of heaviness in the scrotum
- A dull ache in the groin or lower abdomen
- Dull lower back pain.

It is appropriate to seek medical advice if there is a change in the geography of the testes or symptoms appear.

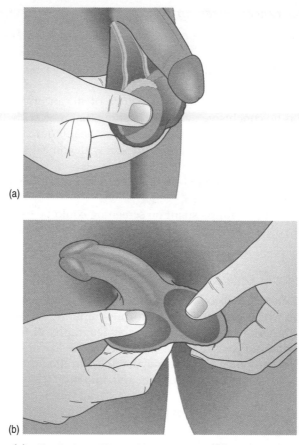

(a)

(b)

Figure 2.2(a) Testicular self examination step 1. **(b)** Testicular self examination step 2.

Routine screening

Austoker (1995, p. 315) states 'Screening for cancer should not be offered routinely to asymptomatic people on a population basis unless it has been shown to be effective in reducing mortality in randomized controlled trials'. Tables 2.5 and 2.6 outline tests that have been shown to be ethical and effective in detecting health problems.

Colorectal cancer

Only 1% of bowel cancers occur in people under 40 years. The risk of bowel cancer increases with age with 99% to the total of this

Table 2.5   Screening physical parameters (Intelihealth)

Parameter	18–39 years	40–49 years	50–64 years	65 years >
Body mass index	3–5 years	1–2 years	annually	annually
Blood pressure	per visit or annually	per visit or annually	per visit or annually	per visit or annually
Serum cholesterol	5 yearly	5 yearly	5 yearly	5 yearly

Table 2.6   Screening for diseases

Disease	18–39 years	40–49 years	50–64 years	65 years >
Prostate cancer		not recommended[a]	not recommended[a]	not recommended[a]
Colorectal cancer			Annual faecal occult blood test (FOBT), sigmoidoscopy (5 yearly), colonoscopy (every 10 years)	Annual faecal occult blood test (FOBT), sigmoidoscopy (5 yearly), colonoscopy (every 10 years)
Diabetes mellitus	every 3 years/ if at risk	every 3 years/ if at risk	every 3 years/ if at risk	every 3 years/ if at risk

[a]Screening for prostate cancer is not recommended in many countries because the tests currently used are not reliable or they carry a high rate of recording a false positive result.

cancer occurring in people over 40 years and 85% occurring in people over 60 years (Hobbs 2000). The rate of colorectal cancer in men is 1 in 18 and for women it is 1 in 20 (Cancer Research UK 2004). Up to 20% of colorectal cancers are thought to have a genetic component (McGrath & Spigelman 2002).

Colorectal cancer commonly evolves slowly from premalignant polyps, indicating an opportunity for early detection and possible removal of polyps. Well-designed prospective randomised trials and case controlled studies have supported the use of screening and the prevention of cancer by removal of polyps. Screening has been found to be cost effective. Screening with faecal occult blood testing reduces mortality of colorectal cancer by approximately 15%.

Delays in diagnosis are caused by:

- Delays in patient seeking help with symptoms
- Delay in referral by the GP to specialists
- Delays by hospitals in establishing diagnosis and timely treatment (Hobbs 2000).

Symptoms

- Persistent rectal bleeding without anal symptoms
- Change in bowel habits (frequency and softer stools)
- Severe anaemia
- Distended abdomen (associated with obstruction).

Many bowel symptoms appear late in the disease process.

Signs

- Palpable abdominal mass
- Palpable rectal mass
- Severe anaemia < 110 g/L in men (secondary sign).

Investigation

- Flexible colonoscopy
- Barium enema.

Prognosis

The prognosis for colorectal cancer is directly related to the time of diagnosis to treatment, therefore early detection is essential. Nearly 80% of cases can be successfully treated if caught at an early stage.

Screening

In the US, colorectal cancer screening is now considered the standard of care for persons over 50 and its omission by GPs is a frequent source of litigation (Winawer 2003). In 2002 the Secretary of state for Health (UK) announced a commitment to introduce a national bowel-screening programme. Although faecal occult blood testing is an inexpensive and easy method, it has a low sensitivity – with about 40% of cancers missed by a single screen. Unfortunately, symptomatic bleeding generally occurs as a later development in colon cancer suggesting a poorer prognosis.

The American Cancer Society recommends:

- Screening of those over 50 years for adenomatous polyps and colorectal cancer.
- Screening of those < 50 years if a familial history of colon cancer exists (first relative, e.g. brother/sister).
- Screening for those who had a relative diagnosed with colon cancer before 60 years.
- Genetic counselling for those patients tested for genetic predisposition to colon cancers.

Screening regimes for those over 50 include:

- Annual faecal occult blood testing (FOBT)
- Flexible sigmoidoscopy every 5 years (combined with FOBT)
- Flexible colonoscopy (every 10 years)
- Barium enema every 5 years (test has a low sensitivity).

For a synopsis of variations in screening regimes refer to Winawer's (2003) report on guidelines.

Screening for depression

Depression is often overlooked and undertreated. There is insufficient evidence to recommend routine screening of children and adolescents for depression; this is despite a prevalence of 2% in children and 4.5% in adolescence. The US Preventative Services Task Force does, however, urge doctors to screen all adult patients for depression (Josefson 2002). Research is ongoing to identify a screening questionnaire that has a high specificity.

References

Action on Smoking and Health (ASH) 2004 Smoking, sex and reproduction. ASH fact sheet No 7 (www.ash.org.uk)

Action on Smoking and Health (ASH) 2005 Smoking statistics: who smokes and how much? ASH fact sheet No 1 (http://www.ash.org.uk/)

Anderson D 1983 Health promotion: an overview. WHO Technical Paper. WHO Regional Office for Europe, Copenhagen

Austoker J 1995 Cancer prevention in primary care: screening for ovarian, prostatic and testicular cancer. British Medical Journal 309(6950): 315–320

Australian Institute of Health and Welfare (AIHW) 2003a Risk Factors: overweight and obesity. Online. Available: http://www.aihw.gov.au/riskfactors/overweight.html

Baldwin B 1979 Gerontological psychiatric nursing. In: Stuart GW, Sundeen SJ Principles and practice of psychiatric nursing. Philadelphia

Baum F 2002 The new public health. Oxford University Press, Melbourne

Berland GK 2001 Commentary. 'With just one click': online health information is abundant, but can it be trusted? [Commentary] Western Journal of Medicine 175(6): 391

British Medical Association 2004 The impact of smoking on sexual, reproductive and child health. Board of Science and Education and Tobacco Control Resource Centre, BMA Publications Unit, London

Brock AC, Griffiths C 2003 Trends in the mortality of young adults aged 15–44 in England and Wales, 1961 to 2001. Health Statistics Quarterly 19(27): 22–31

Cancer Research UK 2004 CancerStats Monograph 2004 – Cancer incidence, survival and mortality in the UK and EU. Cancer Research UK. Online. Available: Cancerstats@cancer.org.uk

Degenhardt L, Hall W, Teesson M et al 2000 Alcohol use disorder in Australia: findings from the National Survey of Mental Health and Well-being, National Drug and Alcohol Research Centre. University of New South Wales, Randwick, Sydney (Technical report 97)

Department of Health 2001 The government response to the Advisory Council on the Misuse of Drugs Report into drug related deaths 2001. The Stationery Office, London

Department of Health 2002 National alcohol harm reduction strategy: consultation document. Joint consultation by the Department of Health and the Cabinet Office to inform work on the National Alcohol Harm Reduction Strategy. The Stationery Office, London. Online. Available: http://www.dh.gov.uk/PublicationsAnd Statistics/Publications/Publications PolicyAndGuidance/PublicationsPolicyAndGuidanceArticle/fs/ en?CONTENT ID=4003162&chk=Xp9K21

Department of Health 2003 Statistical bulletin 2003/20. Statistics on alcohol: England, 2003. Online. Available: http://www.doh.gov.uk/public/sb0320.htm

Department of Health, National Institute for Mental Health in England (DH, NIMHE) 2005 National suicide prevention strategy for England: annual report on progress 2004. The Stationery Office, London. Online. Available: http://www.dh.gov.uk/Publications AndStatistics/Publications/ AnnualReports/ DHAnnualReportsArticle/fs/ en?CONTENT ID=4101668&chk=ZALnoC

Fletcher R, Higginbotham N 2001 Men's perceived health needs. New South Wales Public Health Bulletin 12(12): 327–329

Harris T, Cook EF, Kannel WB et al 1988 Proportional hazards analysis of risk factors for coronary heart disease in individuals aged 65 and older: the Framingham Heart Study. Journal of The American Geriatrics Society 36: 1023–1028

Health Development Agency (HDA) 2002 Cancer prevention: a resource to support local action in delivering the NHS cancer plan. Chapter 5 Alcohol. Addressing alcohol misuse: strategic aims. Online. Available: http://www.hda-online.org.uk/html/resources/cancerprevention/introduction.html

Hirst G, Ward J, Del Mar C 1996 Prostate cancer screening: the case against. Medical Journal of Australia 164: 285–287

Hobbs R 2000 ABC of colorectal cancer: the role of primary care. British Medical Journal 321(7268): 1068–1070

Intelihealth Screening for men. Medical content reviewed by the faculty of the Harvard Medical School. Online. Available: http://www.intelihealth.com/IH/ihtIH

Josefson D 2002 US task force recommends screening for depression. British Medical Journal 324(7349): 1293

Laws TA, Drummond M, Poljak-Fligic J 2000 On what basis do Australian men make informed decisions about diagnostic and treatment options for prostate cancer? Australian Journal of Primary Health Interchange 6(2): 86–93

McGrath DR, Spigelman AD 2002 Hereditary colorectal cancer: keeping it in the family – the bowel cancer story. Internal Medical Journal 32(7): 325–330

National Drug and Alcohol Research Centre (NDARC) 2003 Guidelines for treatment of alcohol problems. National alcohol strategy. Australian Government Department of Health and Ageing

National Health and Medical Research Council (NHMRC) 2001 Australian alcohol guidelines: health risks and benefits. Commonwealth of Australia. ACT, Canberra. Online. Available: http://www.nhmrc.gov.au/publications/pdf/ds9.pdf

National Screening Committee 1998 First report of the National Screening Committee, National Screening Committee, Health Departments of the United Kingdom

New South Wales Department of Health 2000 Alcohol and other drugs. Policy for nursing practice in NSW: a framework for progress 2000–2003. Better Health Centre Publications Warehouse, Gladesville, Australia

Punglia RS, D'Amico AV, Catalona MD et al 2003 Effect of verification bias on screening for prostate cancer by measurement of prostate-specific antigen. The New England Journal of Medicine 349(4): 335–342

QUIT 2005 Tobacco in Australia: facts and issues, trends in tobacco consumption. The Cancer Council, Victoria, Australia. Online. Available: http://www.quit.org.au/quit/FandI/welcome.htm

Raffle AE, Alden B, Quinn M et al 2003 Outcomes of screening to prevent cancer: analysis of cumulative incidence of cervical abnormality and modelling of cases and deaths prevented. British Medical Journal 326(7395): 901–906

Simpura J, Karlsson T 2001 Trends in drinking patterns in fifteen European countries, 1950 to 2000. A collection of country reports. STAKES, Helsinki

Sladden M, Dickinson J 1993 Effectiveness of screening for prostate cancer. Australian Family Physician 22(8): 1385–1392

Taylor JS 1993 Carcinoma of the prostate. Medical Journal of Australia 159(7): 436–437

Tong S, Hughes K, Oldenburg B et al 2004 Would general practitioners support a population-based colorectal cancer screening programme of faecal-occult blood testing? Internal Medicine Journal 34(9–10): 532–538

Wicke DM, Lorge RE, Coppin RJ et al 1994 The effectiveness of waiting room notice boards as a vehicle for health education. Family Practice 11: 292–295

Winawer SJ 2003 New colorectal cancer screening guidelines: a consensus for action. British Medical Journal 327(7408): 196–197

World Health Organisation 1978 International Conference on Primary Health Care, Alma-Ata, USSR. WHO Regional Office for Europe, Copenhagen. Online. Available: http://www.who.dk/AboutWHO/Policy/200108252

World Health Organisation 1986 Ottawa Charter for health promotion. Document endorsed by the First International Conference on Health Promotion. WHO, Ottawa

World Health Organisation Working Group 1995 Alcohol and health – implications for public health policy. Report of a WHO Working Group, Oslo

Further reading

Enoch MA 2002 How can I help my patient stop drinking? American Family Physician 65(7): 1475–1476

Enoch MA, Goldman D 2002 Problem drinking and alcoholism: diagnosis and treatment. ACT, Canberra 65(3): 441–448

Fisher K, Howat PA, Binns CW et al 1986 Health education and health promotion: an Australian perspective. Health Education Journal 45(2): 95–98

NHMRC 2001 Australian alcohol guidelines: health risks and benefits. Commonwealth of Australia. American Family Physician (reprinted 2003). http://www.nhmrc.gov.au/publications/pdf/ds9.pdf

Stewart KB, Richards AB 2000 Recognizing and managing your patient's alcohol abuse. Nursing 30(3): 56–59

Resources: health promotion websites

American Public Health Association (APHA) http://www.apha.org/

Canadian Public Health Association http://www.cpha.ca

Declaration of Alma-Ata can be gained by typing 'Alma-Ata' into most search engines. Many universities have copies on their web site (e.g. University of Queensland). http://www.sph.uq.edu.au/cphc/phc/almaata.html

Department of Health – Public Health & Clinical Quality with NHS links. www.doh.gov.uk/publich.htm

Health Education Board for Scotland http://www.hebs.scot.nhs.uk/

NHS Health Development Agency (HDA) http://www.hda-online.org.uk/

New South Wales Health: Health Promotion Branch http://www.health.nsw.gov.au/public-health/health-promotion/abouthp/links.html

Chapter 3

Ethico-legal issues

IMPLICATIONS FOR PRACTICE

Nurses need an understanding of current legislature in their geographical area of practice as well as knowledge of developments in regions and countries similar to their own. This knowledge is the basis for practising in a way that minimises complaints and litigious actions by clients and patients. Knowledge of the law also aids in the promotion of the rights of individuals and communities through scholarly debate and submissions to professional bodies.

SURROGACY BY IN VITRO FERTILISATION

Men who intend to become fathers through surrogacy should be aware of the legal and ethical implications. More than 300 births, from natural and in vitro fertilisation surrogacy arrangements, have occurred in Britain. In vitro fertilisation involves the genetic parents donating both sets of gametes. The woman receiving the embryos created from the gametes of the genetic couple is known as the surrogate host. The following should be borne in mind:

- Treatment of the commissioning couple and the host must be done in clinics licensed by the Human Fertilisation and Embryology Authority United Kingdom.
- Review of each surrogacy arrangement by an independent ethics committee is strongly recommended.
- In-depth counselling is essential for the preparation of couples for treatment.

Complications

Complications of treatment are minimal with appropriate selection and counselling. However, surrogacy arrangements sometimes result in unreasonably high expectations of success, in spite of frank information and counselling. For example, failure to conceive a pregnancy often causes severe stress for all parties, with the host feeling guilty that she has lost the genetic couple's chance of a child and the genetic couple feeling guilt because of the stress associated with miscarriage. The host must also cope with the need for dilation and curettage (Brinsden et al 2000).

Legalities

The Human Fertilisation and Embryology Act 1990 (section 36) declares surrogacy contracts as 'unenforceable' in law. The Act defines the child's legal mother as the woman completing the pregnancy, regardless of whether mother and child are genetically related (section 27). Sections 27 and 30 ensure that if the surrogate host decides to keep the child she is legally entitled to do so. If the commissioning couple reject the child then it remains the legal responsibility of the host.

Paternity

Under section 30 of the 1990 Act, the commissioning couple are not required to apply for adoption of the child and may receive 'parental orders' if they have the consent of the birth mother and are:

- married
- over 18
- genetically related to the child (one or both)
- domiciled in the UK, Channel Islands, or Isle of Man

- already caring for the child
- not paying the birth mother more than reasonable expenses.

N. B. The application must be made *within 6 months* of the birth of the child.

REPRODUCTIVE RIGHTS

Fatherhood and paternity

Advances in reproductive technology have opened up new opportunities for those unable to have children in the usual way. However, substantial legal and ethical dilemmas arise concerning men and fatherhood. The following examples have been taken from media coverage and medical papers and are intended to demonstrate the complexity of the issues surrounding paternity rights:

- Couples can now, with the aid of science, create a frozen embryo. The salient question is who owns that embryo. Two women have recently gone to court to secure their rights to embryos created by themselves and their now ex-partners. These men, who are the biological fathers, want the embryos destroyed (case pending).
- Recently, homosexual men in Britain were legally allowed to become surrogate parents. Is there any evidence to show that homosexual couples (gay or lesbians) do not make good parents or that the children in these families are less emotionally/psychologically adjusted than other children?
- A black man who donated sperm to a fertility clinic had his sperm incorrectly allocated to a white couple during an in vitro fertilisation procedure. He was declared the legal father in a High Court decision (Dyer 2003).
- Should men have a right to choose whether or not a pregnancy should go ahead? This question is premised on the fact that half of the genetic material in an embryo belongs to the father. This type of claim may be perceived as another means of men exerting power over women.
- The media have highlighted several cases where fathers have been making child support payments to the mother when they are not the biological father. A simple swab of the child's mouth can be used to map and find a match with paternal genes. This practice has prompted concerns about privacy and in some countries it is now illegal. However, web based access to US laboratories with questionable protocols continue to be used.

- A man was bludgeoned to death by a police officer in New York. In the morgue his widow asked the medical-examiner to extract his sperm so she could bear his child. The medical-examiner contacted the hospital's fertility unit (Bauman 1997).
- The High Court has ruled that the Home Secretary has the power not to assist prisoners in begetting children whilst they are serving a jail sentence.
- A Californian teenager in 2003 became the first sperm bank baby to meet her biological father under new rules in the US that allowed the release of the father's identity.

Nursing issues

The points just covered emphasise the need for nurses to understand the law and the current state of play of ethical practice, particularly in relation to reproductive technology. This can be achieved by:

- Requesting staff development sessions from in-house presenters or guest speakers from specialist organisations.
- Attending conferences where ethical and legal aspects of reproductive practice are tabled.
- Accessing journals that have a special section in each edition on ethical issues.
- Engaging in debate/discussion with other health professionals and nursing colleagues about a case or a hypothetical situation. This allows the professional to explore current or proposed practice vis-à-vis professional codes of ethics.

Given that scientific developments usually precede a comprehensive evaluation of the legal and ethical implications, the activities listed here represent a very useful means of coming to terms with personal values and beliefs as well as being prepared for issues in clinical practice.

HOMOSEXUALITY

The term homosexuality is a medical one and it is used in law and medical science to denote deviancy from heterosexuality. This claim is evidenced by the classifications used in the *ICD-9* (World Health Organisations). However, men who have sexual relationships with other men prefer to be referred to as 'gay' and see their sexual preference as normal.

Medical classification of sexual deviations and disorders

This classification comes under the section 'Mental Disorders' (290–319) in the World Health Organisation's ICD-9-CM.

302 sexual deviations and disorders
302.0 Homosexuality
302.1 Zoophilia
302.2 Pedophilia
302.3 Transvestism
302.4 Exhibitionism
302.5 Trans-sexualism
302.6 Disorders of psychosexual identity
302.7 Psychosexual dysfunction
302.8 Other specified psychosexual disorders
302.9 Unspecified psychosexual disorder

Ethical issues

There is systemic and widespread discrimination faced by those who are identified with or identified as non-heterosexuals. Moreover, discrimination on the grounds of homosexuality in the areas of employment, education, accommodation, and the provision of goods, services and other facilities is widespread in society yet often against the law (Kendall 1996).

The British Medical Association Equal Opportunities Committee (2003) reports that:

Discrimination on the grounds of sexual orientation is not currently prohibited per se by the SDA [Sex Discrimination Act] 1975. As the law currently stands, to prove discrimination a homosexual male employee would have to prove that he has suffered less favourable treatment, by reason of his sexual orientation, than a female homosexual experienced in a similar position to him, or vice versa. If a female homosexual has been subjected to similar treatment, no discrimination would arise under the SDA. Individuals may also be able to gain some protection under Article 8 of the Human Rights Act 1998, which provides the right to respect for private and family life.

In an effort to minimise discrimination and promote equality new legislation has been enacted in many countries. There is recognition that:

- Gay men may hold key religious positions
- Men in a gay relationship should hold the same rights as married couples
- Young people should be taught about variances in sexuality as a means of reducing homophobia
- Gay men who have children should be able to adopt those children into a gay relationship.

Military law and regulations

Military law and regulations state that medical doctors and other health personnel have a duty to inform their commanding officer if a member of the forces is known to be homosexual. However, the British Medical Association (BMA) does not consider that sexual orientation, without other indicators of a risk to others, is sufficient cause to require such reporting. Moreover, two European Court of Human Rights judgments have ruled that the discharge of personnel from the UK armed forces solely on grounds of their homosexuality contravenes Article 8 of the 1950 European Convention for the Protection of Human Rights and Fundamental Freedoms. As a result of a challenge in the European Court of Human Rights in 1999, new guidance may emerge for armed forces' doctors in respect of the duty to report homosexuality (BMA 1999).

Same sex relationships

Over the past decade many countries, including Britain, France, South Africa, Hungary, Iceland and the USA have moved to enact legal recognition of same sex relationships. The Civil Partnership Act (UK) (2004) allows homosexual couples to sign a document giving them the same rights and responsibilities as their married counterparts. An internet version of the Act is published by the Queen's Printer of Acts of Parliament and has been prepared to reflect the text as it received Royal Assent (http://www.publications.parliament.uk/pa/ld200304/labills/053/2004053.htm). Couples will be able to receive:

- A joint treatment for income-related benefits
- Joint pension benefits
- An ability to gain parental responsibility for each other's children
- Recognition for immigration purposes

- Exemption from testifying against each other in court
- Benefit from a dead partner's pension
- Next of kin rights in hospitals
- Exemption from inheritance tax on a dead partner's home
- Dissolution of an agreement similar to that of divorce.

In Australia at this time there is no indication that the Howard government intends to remove legislative discrimination against people in a same sex relationship. However, the state of Tasmania is the first Australian state to set up a registry of same sex relationships. The registry will allow same sex couples to adopt where one of the partners is a parent of the child.

Age of consent

The age of consent for a sexual relationship between a male and female is clearly defined in law but differs between countries, states and regions. Similar age differentials exist in relation to homosexual relations between men. However, in many countries across Europe the age of consent is higher for homosexuals. Calls for law reform in this area are based on the notion that differential age of consent laws discriminate against gay men (British Medical Association Equal Opportunities Committee 2003).

There is no overarching legislation that defines the age of consent in Australia. Each state and territory has its own legislation with some stating 14 years of age and others guided by the Gillick case (1986) (see Box 3.1).

Box 3.1   The Gillick case

The Department of Health and Social Security issued a circular containing advice to the effect that a doctor could consult about contraception with a girl under the age of 16 years without parental consent. Although he should try to persuade the girl to involve her parents in the matter, the principle of confidentiality between doctor and patient was a primary tenet. When the authority refused to give an assurance to the parents that they would be informed if their daughter was to be given such advice the plaintiff brought an action against the

Box 3.1   The Gillick case—cont'd

authority and the department. Initially the decision was in the plaintiff's favour. Eventually, the Department appealed to the House of Lords. Lord Templeman's review included the following points:

Having regard to the reality that a child became increasingly independent as it grew older and that parental authority dwindled correspondingly, the law did not recognise any rule of absolute parental authority until a fixed age. Instead, parental rights were recognised by the law only as long as they were needed for the protection of the child and such rights yielded to the child's right to make his own decisions when he reached a sufficient understanding and intelligence to be capable of making up his own mind.

Accordingly, a girl under 16 did not, merely by reason of her age, lack legal capacity to consent to contraceptive advice and treatment by a doctor. (Gillick v. West Norfolk and Wisbech Area Health Authority http://www.hrcr.org/safrica/childrens_rights/Gillick_WestNorfolk.htm)

In many countries across Europe the age of consent is higher for homosexuals than heterosexuals. Calls for law reform in this area are based on the notion that differential age of consent laws discriminate against gay men (British Medical Association 2003). An insight into the debates surrounding an equitable age of consent can gleaned from a 1994 report produced by the British Medical Association (see website reference). In England, the Age of Consent Sexual Offences (Amendment) Bill received royal assent and eventually made law on 30th November 2000. The age of consent is now 16 years, irrespective of sexual orientation.

Teaching about homosexuality

In Scotland teachers have been able to inform students about homosexuality for some years. However, in England Section 28 (see below) prevented such teachings. Teaching young people only about heterosexual relationships does little to minimise the stigma attached to homosexuality.

Homophobia

Sexual health issues

Studies identifying forms of masculinity that gain the most respect in society have concluded that there is an almost compulsory heterosexuality and concomitant homophobia. Consequently, school boys and adolescents are likely to be victimised if they show homosexual tendencies or fraternise with known homosexuals. Where family members express negative emotions towards gay men, the young men in these families may feel that they would be victimised if they disclose that they are not heterosexual (disclosure of homosexuality is referred to as coming out). In public life professional bodies, such as the British Medical Association have policies (British Medical Association 2003) designed to ensure that all members, those applying for membership, and other service users will receive the highest possible standards of service, irrespective of race, ethnicity, gender and sexual orientation. The Royal College of Nursing (2002, p. 3) also notes that in:

> 'Smith v Gardner Merchant (1999) ICR 135: the court of appeal held that discrimination on the grounds of sexual orientation does not fall within the Sex Discrimination Act. However it did decide that it was unlawful sex discrimination to treat a homosexual less favourably than a female lesbian.'

In the case of McDonald versus Ministry of Defence (1998) IRLR 'the Scottish Appeal Tribunal held that there was discrimination on the grounds of sexual orientation under the Sex Discrimination Act.'

Effects of discrimination/victimisation

A consequence of legal discrimination, denigration and victimisation is a sense of fear and low self-esteem. A lowered sense of self-esteem among gay men, in response to discrimination, denigration and victimisation, has been reported as leading to:

- Illicit drug use
- Depression
- Alcohol use

- Increased rates of attempted suicide (though this varies between regions).

Epidemiological studies from North America and New Zealand show that gay and bisexual males are at least four times as likely to report serious attempts at suicide (Bagley & D'Augelli 2000).

Reducing homophobia

Section 28 of the Local Government Act, 1988, introduced by Margaret Thatcher's government banning the promotion of homosexuality by councils stated that: 'A local authority shall not (a) intentionally promote homosexuality or publish material with the intention of promoting homosexuality; (b) promote the teaching in any maintained school of the acceptability of homosexuality as a pretended family relationship.'

Section 28 prohibited the teaching of sexuality outside that of heterosexual relations. Although the Act was finally repealed with effect from 18 November 2003 by Section 122 of the Local Government Act 2003 (enacted on 18 September 2003), many schools provide no strategies to minimise homophobia. Consequently, school nurses will have an important role as confidants to those boys wanting to discuss sexual issues or declaring that their wellbeing is affected by victimisation based on sexual issues.

Nursing issues

Consider the following questions as having important implications for your practice:

- Are gay men treated any differently in your area of health service? If so, why?
- Are staff showing negative attitudes to gay men (by verbalising stereotypes, avoiding contact with these men or displaying negative body language)?
- How are sexual relations documented in case notes and what are their legal implication (e.g. enduring power of attorney/next of kin)?
- Have there been staff development updates regarding the implications for practice relating to changes in the law concerning gay men?

Reflective exercise

List the words that come to mind when the following terms are used:

- Homosexual
- Gay men
- Lesbian
- Heterosexual couples.

Mark next to each word a tick for positive and a cross for negative connotations/perceptions. Identify the ways you have been exposed to the negative connotations that you have attached to the sexualities listed (e.g. media, friends, health services). Explore why you hold negative perceptions and what you seek to achieve by continuing to support these perceptions in your practice.

References

Age of Consent Sexual Offences (Amendment) Act 2000 The Stationery Office, London

Bagley C, D'Augelli AR 2000 Suicidal behaviour in gay, lesbian and bisexual youth. British Medical Journal 320(7250): 1617–1618

Bauman N 1997 Dead men conceiving: trend raises ethical, legal questions. Urology Times 25(2)

Brindsden PR, Appleton TC, Murray E et al 2000 Treatment by in vitro fertilisation with surrogacy: experience of one British centre. British Medical Journal 320(7239): 924–929

British Medical Association 1994 Age of consent for homosexual men: a scientific and medical perspective. Online. Available: http://www.geocities.com/richardg_uk/bma.html

British Medical Association 1999 Confidentiality and disclosure of health information. Online. Available: http://www.bma.org.uk/ap.nsf/Content/BibliographyofrelevantBMApubl

British Medical Association Equal Opportunities Commission 2003 Dealing with discrimination: guidelines for BMA members. Online. Available: http://www.bma.org.uk/ap.nsf/Content/discrimination?OpenDocument&Highlight=2,homosexual

Civil Partnership Act 2004 The Stationery Office, London

Dyer C 2003 Biological father declared the legal father in IVF mix up. British Medical Journal 326(7388): 518

Gillick v West Norfolk and Wisbech Area Health Authority 1986 House of Lords [1986] 1 AC 112 [1985] 3 All ER 402, [1985] 3 WLR 830, [1986] 1 FLR 224, [1986] Crim LR 113, 2 BMLR 11

Human Fertilisation and Embryology Act 1990 HMSO, London
Kendall C 1996 Homophobia as an issue of sex discrimination: lesbian and gay
  equality and the systemic effects of forced invisibility. Murdoch University
  Electronic Journal of Law 3(3). Online. Available:
  http://www.murdoch.edu.au/elaw/issues/v3n3/kendall.html
Local Government Act 2003 The Stationery Office, London
Royal College of Nursing 2002 Challenging harassment and bullying: working
  well initiative: guidance for RCN representatives, stewards and officers.
  Royal College of Nursing, London. Online. Available:
  http://www.rcn.org.uk/publications/pdf/Challenging%20Bullying%20-%
  20Reps%20guide.pdf
World Health Organisation/National Register of Hospital Statistics (NRHS)
  International classification of diseases, 9th revision, clinical modification
  (ICD-9-CM). WHO, Geneva. Online. Available:
  http://www.newcastle.edu.au/centre/hsrg/hypertexts/icd9cm.html

Further reading

British Medical Association 1996 Changing conceptions of motherhood – the
  practice of surrogacy in Britain. BMA Professional Division Publications
Rivers L 2004 Recollections of bullying at school and their long-term implications
  for lesbians, gay men, and bisexuals. Crisis 25(4): 169–175
Rondahl G, Innala S, Carlsson M 2004 Nursing staff and nursing students' emo-
  tions towards homosexual patients and their wish to refrain from nursing, if
  the option existed. Scandinavian Journal of Caring Sciences 18(1): 19–26
Smith AM, Rissel CE, Richters J et al 2003 Sex in Australia: sexual identity, sexual
  attraction and sexual experience among a representative sample of adults.
  Australian and New Zealand Journal of Public Health 27(2): 138–145
Tate FB, Longo DA 2004 Homophobia: a challenge for psychosocial nursing.
  Journal of Psychosocial Nursing and Mental Health Services 42(8): 26–33

Resources

*Information regarding legal recognition of same sex relationships around Australia, pre-
pared by the Let's Get Equal Campaign Working Party is available online at:*
http://www.aidscouncil.org.au/equalinfo.htm

Chapter **4**

Young men

PREMATURE DEATHS

What kills young males?

Even though only 5% of total UK deaths occur among young adults, a third of these are attributable to accidental injury, self inflicted injury and poisoning and are therefore considered 'avoidable'. Other statistics include:

- From the 1990s suicide has become more common (see Chapter 1). Suicide notes left by young men often mention depression and poor health as a reason for suicide (O'Connor & Sheehy 2000, p. 79).
- Alcohol related mortality has risen, in young adult males and females, to the extent that it has almost tripled from 1979 to 2001.
- Death from drug-related poisoning for young people tripled between 1979 and 2001 to a rate of 13% in young males and 7% in young females (Brock & Griffiths 2003).

Overall, between 1985 and 2001 the death rate (all causes) has increased by 193% in young men, compared with 40% for young women (Brock & Griffiths 2003).

SUBSTANCE ABUSE

Deaths attributable to accidental poisoning, drug dependence and drug abuse accounted for approximately 6% of all deaths for young adult males in the 1980s. In the 1990s drug related mortality for men grew at a rate three times that of women.

Between 1985 and 2001 the overall death rate increased by 193% in young men and 40% in young women (Brock & Griffiths 2003).

Trends in drug abuse fatalities: 1997–1999

- Suicide by drug poisoning was up by two thirds.
- Accidental poisoning increased three-fold.
- Drug dependence was up four-fold.

Cause of fatal poisoning (see Table 4.1)

- In 1993 methadone featured most on death certificates.
- In 2001 heroin/morphine featured most on death certificates.

TEENAGE BOYS DRINKING

In 2002, about a quarter (24%) of pupils in England aged 11–15 years had drunk alcohol in the previous week. The proportion of

Table 4.1 Most frequently mentioned substance appearing on drug-related poisoning death certificates (Office of National Statistics (UK) 2001)

Substance	Number of men	% of drug related poisoning
Heroin/morphine	717	47.0
Methadone	151	9.9
Benzodiazepines	133	8.7
All antidepressants	129	8.5
Paracetamol (including compounds)	109	7.1
All amphetamines	61	4.0
TOTAL drug-poisoning deaths	1526	

students drinking has fluctuated round about this level since the mid 1990s (DH 2001).

Modifying drinking

Research commissioned by the Australian government showed that parents are openly looking for help in dealing with their teenagers and drinking. At the same time, many teenagers are clearly looking to their parents to set some boundaries about alcohol.

Encouraging parents to talk with their teenagers about alcohol is one of the aims in the next phase of Australia's National Alcohol Campaign. The campaign is designed to help young Australians think about the choices they make about drinking and turn around the growing number of young Australians who are consuming alcohol excessively. The campaign targets teenagers aged 15–17 years, with secondary target audiences of parents of 12–17 year olds and young people aged 18–24 years. Campaign materials are accessible on-line (www.nationalalcoholcampaign.health.gov.au) (Australian Government Media Release 2002).

N. B. See Chapter 2 Promoting health for alcohol assessment strategies and health promotion interventions.

BODY IMAGE

The commodification of women's bodies by various forms of media has been starkly evident over the past few decades and now it seems there is a similar focus on young men's bodies, with commensurate social pressures. At times these pressures give rise to substantial physical and psychological health problems.

Self-appraisal of body image occurs mostly through a social comparison of personal attributes (body size, shape and general appearance) with those of idealised media images and peer group norms. Repeated exposure to media images of *muscular males* and *thin females* make these body forms appear to be the standard for an attractive body image. Young men seeking to attain a muscular image have turned to steroid use. Pope et al (2000) note that an estimated 6–7% of high school boys have used these drugs. Neumark-Sztainer et al (1999) found 2.3% of boys using steroids over a period compared to 0.5% of females. Youth from the 'low' socioeconomic groups who had issues about their body image were at greater risk of developing an eating disorder.

> **Key points**
>
> - The pressure on boys and men to mimic a socially idealised male body image (muscular and lean) is increasing.
> - Same sex peer teasing among boys made self-evaluation of *weight* more critical.
> - Dissatisfaction with body image almost certainly contributes to the development of low self-esteem, depression and body image disorders (Jones 2002).
> - Concerns about body image may lead to social isolation and depression.
> - Several studies in the US indicate that high school boys take anabolic steroids to enhance body muscularity, shape and size.

Body dysmorphic disorder (BDD)

Although women have traditionally had more cultural constraints placed on their body shape and size, there are now suggestions that men are increasingly concerned with their body image and appearance. An American study identified 43% of men as being dissatisfied with their overall appearance (Pope et al 2000). This figure represents a three-fold increase in dissatisfaction over a 25 year period and indicates that nearly as many men as women are now dissatisfied with how they look. Severe forms of self-preoccupation with *body image* can result in a pathological psychiatric disorder termed body dysmorphic disorder (BDD) or dysmorphobia. Men and boys with body image problems do not recognise that their beliefs about their appearance are inaccurate and the true extent of BDD remains hidden because men are reluctant to disclose they have a problem.

Characteristics of men with BDD

- They are overtly occupied with examining their external features
- Nearly all perform repetitive behaviours directed towards identifying personal physical defects (e.g. nose size and shape, genital size and skin blemishes).
- They spend an inordinate amount of time attempting to hide perceived defects.

- Despite the use of dermatological and surgical remedies many men remain dissatisfied with their image after treatment and as a consequence can become severely depressed, even suicidal (Phillips & Castle 2001).
- Teasing about physical attributes by peers may trigger BDD.
- A preoccupation with an imagined deficit or defect in appearance can cause clinically significant distress interfering with job performance.
- Concerns about body image may lead to social isolation and depression (Drummond 1999, 2001).

Eating disorders

Linking body image and eating disorders

Whilst there is information that explores femininity/feminism in relation to weight loss, there is only emerging research concerned with analysing body image, masculinity and health (Drummond 1999). Eating disorders are perceived by society as a female disorder, consequently, men with this diagnosis experience it as an affront to their masculinity.

Forms of eating disorders

The two most commonly diagnosed forms of eating disorders are **anorexia nervosa and bulimia nervosa.** Anorexia nervosa is characterised by a refusal to maintain a minimum normal body weight, by means of dietary restrictions, fasting and often self-induced vomiting and purging. Bulimia nervosa is characterised by repeated episodes of binge eating followed by self-induced vomiting, inappropriate use of laxatives or enemas, fasting and excessive exercise (AMA 1994). Both forms of eating disorders are directed towards avoiding weight gain; as such, many clinicians argue that the two disorders lie on a continuum.

Prevalence of eating disorders

Based on the number of individuals who seek assistance from healthcare professionals for eating disorders, Drewnowski and Yee (1987) estimate the prevalence of eating disorders among men is between 5 and 10%. In a study of adolescent Americans Neumark-Sztainer et al (1999) found that behaviours related to eating disorders (vomiting, use of diet pills, laxatives and diuretics) occurred in

7.4% of girls and 3.1% of boys in the week preceding the survey. Striegel et al (1999), in a study of war veterans, found the incidence of eating disorders to be 3.0% among 24 041 women and 0.02% among 466.590 men. Whilst the figures for men are substantially less in magnitude than for women with similar eating problems, it is argued that men may be under-represented (Pope et al 2000) because:

- men in general are less likely to use health services
- men with an eating disorder perceive the disorder to be a feminised illness and try to hide their difficulties
- the humiliation men feel from exhibiting signs of an eating disorder makes them reticent to approach health services.

Consequently, male eating disorders are not yet perceived as 'a serious public health issue' (Drummond 1999).

Causes of eating disorders in men

In reviewing the causes of eating disorders among men, it is important to note that the way masculinity is socially constructed plays an important part in their manifestation and management. Research shows that eating disorders are often present in the pre-adolescent period, yet little is known about the onset of these disorders and associated risk factors. In the case of children Schur et al's (2000) survey of boys and girls revealed that 50% of all children wanted to lose weight. Edmunds and Hill (1999), in their study of 2000 girls and 202 boys aged 12 years, found that parents played an active role in their children's dieting. Fasting and dietary restraint were found among 20% of girls and 8% of boys. Kelly et al (1999) claimed that although dieting in boys is relatively infrequent, emotional concerns about eating were predicted by poorer body image and lower self-esteem. Research is also showing the following:

- Pope et al (2000) have identified that men are increasingly becoming preoccupied with weight and body fat composition.
- Issues of competitiveness feature strongly in interviews with men who have an eating disorder; they either compete to be the thinnest or compete to appear the sickest in comparison with other males with eating disorders (Drummond 1999).
- Eating disorders associated with anorexia and bulimia nervosa are being found increasingly among male athletes and men (Zerbe 1999).

- The assumption that dieting is a feminine trait deters some men from restrictions on food; more masculine means of weight loss include gruelling exercise regimes, diuretics, purging (dehydration is a dangerous consequence).
- Men with eating disorders were found to have high rates of co-morbid organic mental health problems, schizophrenic/psychotic episodes, substance abuse and mood disorders.

Groups most at risk

Men with eating disorders were found to have:

- higher rates of co-morbid mental health problems and psychotic episodes (e.g. schizophrenic)
- been sexually assaulted
- a family history (for a broad spectrum of eating disorders).

The assumed higher incidence of eating disorders in gay men relative to heterosexual men has not been established. However, heterosexual men are more likely to conceal the problem because they are afraid of been labelled as 'gay'. Men tend not to seek help until the problem is well developed, making successful treatment less likely. Given that there are substantial reasons for men not wanting to disclose they have an eating disorder, nurses should focus on assessment skills that aid in the detection of eating disorders before they become critical (Laws & Drummond 2001).

Nursing issues

Spend some time considering how you might create non-threatening questions for interviewing men with an actual or suspected eating disorder. Uses the categories of:
- Ideal weight
- Image of themselves
- Exercise
- Diet
- Social activities
- Medications/dietary supplements.

Nursing issues

Spend some time summarising, in your mind, how the following assessment items may alert you to the need for further investigation of an eating disorder among males in your health service.

- Blood picture
- BMI
- Mental state assessment (e.g. depression/mood)
- Interview impressions (e.g. self-esteem)
- Behavioural traits (e.g. obsessive)
- At risk groups
- Age groups.

References

American Psychiatric Association 1994 Diagnastic and statistical manual of mental health disorders, 4th edn. American Psychiatric Association, Washington DC

Australian Government Media Release 16 June 2002 Trish Worth MP. Online. Available: http://www.health.gov.au/mediarel/yr 2002/tw/tw02014.htm

Brock AC, Griffiths C 2003 Trends in the mortality of young adults aged 15–44 in England and Wales, 1996–2001. Health Statistics Quarterly 19(27): 22–31.

Department of Health 2001 Statistics on smoking, drinking and drug use among young people in 2000. Ref no 2001/0344. Online. Available: http://www.dh. gov.uk/AdvancedSearch/SearchResults/fs/en?NP=1&PO1-C&PI1-W&PF1-A&PG-1&RP-20&PT1-drinking&SC-dh site&Z-1

Drewnowski A, Yee D 1987 Men and body image: are males satisfied with their body weight? Psychosomatic Medicine 49(6): 626–634

Drummond M 1999 Life as a male anorexic. Australian Journal of Primary Health – Interchange 5(2): 80–89

Drummond M 2001 Boys' bodies in the context of sport and physical activity: implications for health. Journal of Physical Education New Zealand 34(1): 53–64

Edmunds H, Hill AJ 1999 Dieting and the family context of eating in young adolescent children. International Journal of Eating Disorders 25(4): 435–440

Jones CJ 2002 Social comparison and body image: attractiveness comparisons to models and peers among adolescent girls and boys. Sex Roles 9/10: 645–664

Kelly C, Ricciardelli LA, Clarke JD 1999 Problem eating attitudes and behaviours in young children. International Journal of Eating Disorders 25(3): 281–286

Laws TA, Drummond MJ 2001 A proactive approach to assessing men for eating disorders. Contemporary Nurse 11: 28–39

Neumark-Sztainer D, Story M, Falkner NH et al 1999 Sociodemographic and personal characteristics of adolescents engaged in weight loss and weight/muscle gain behaviours: who is doing what? Preventive Medicine 28(1): 40–50

O'Cannor R, Sheehy N 2000 Understanding suicidal behaviour. British Psychological Society/Blackwell, Oxford

Office of National Statistics UK 2005 Deaths 2001: coroner consultation and final method of certification. Mortality statistics, general, 2001 (series DHI no 34). Online. Available: http://www.statistics.gov.uk /STATBASE/ xsdataset.asp?vink-7137&More-Y

Phillips KA, Castle DJ 2001 Body dysmorphic disorder in men. British Medical Journal 323(7320): 1015–1016

Pope H, Phillips K, Olivardia R 2000 The Adonis complex: the secret crisis of male body obsession. The Free Press, New York

Schur EA, Sanders M, Steiner H 2000 Body dissatisfaction and dieting in young children. International Journal of Eating Disorders 27(1): 74–82

Striegel-Moore RH, Garvin V, Dohm F et al 1999 Eating disorders in a national sample of hospitalized female and male veterans: detection rates and psychiatric comorbidity. International Journal of Eating Disorders 25(4): 405–414

Zerbe KJ 1999 Anorexia nervosa and bulimia nervosa: when the pursuit of bodily 'perfection' becomes a killer. Postgraduate Medicine 99(1): 161–164, 167–169, 209–211

Further reading

Halek C 1997 Eating disorders: the role of the nurse. Professional development section. Nursing Times 93(28): 63–65

Love CC, Seaton H 1991 Eating disorders: highlights of nursing assessment and therapeutics. Nursing Clinics of North America 26(3): 677–697

Muscari M 1998 Screening for anorexia and bulimia. America Journal of Nursing 98(11): 22, 24

Chapter 5

Prime time

CHAPTER CONTENTS

The prime focus of this chapter is male reproductive issues because, aside from workplace and employment issues, the quality of sexual relations and being able to father a child are key concerns for men in the prime of their life. The reproductive issues explored in the first part of this chapter are linked to the pathogenesis of reproduction and consequences of infections, problems in achieving pregnancy, family planning and vasectomy. As prime time curtails, men become more concerned about their ability to have and maintain sexual relations. These topics are addressed later in the chapter with reference to biological and psychological problems (e.g. erectile dysfunction and androgen insufficiency).

INFERTILITY AND SUBFERTILITY

Infertility can be generally defined as non pregnancy in a couple who have 'tried for a child' for 1 year. Approximately 10% of couples experience infertility as just defined. About one third of infertilities arise from problems with the male reproductive physiology, with 1:20 men affected by some form of subfertility (Hirsh 2003). Most men with erectile dysfunction or ejaculation failure have normal sperm function. In these cases the challenge is to stimulate ejaculation. Treatment with sindenafil may be useful for those men who are unable to produce a sample of ejaculate (Hirsht, 2003).

Who should assess men's fertility?

- Gynaecologist trained in reproductive medicine
- Clinical andrologist in a reproduction medical clinic.

Diagnosis

Semen analysis takes place at the pathology service or fertility clinic. Reliable results can only be gained if men avoid heavy intake of alcohol and hot saunas/baths, drug treatments and illness prior to donation. Haemochromatosis is well established as a cause of infertility in men and women because iron is deposited in the gonads leading to hypogonadism. Deposition of iron in the pituitary may lead to pituitary dysfunction contributing to hypogonadism (Tweed & Roland 1998).

Significant abnormalities in sperm

These include:

- no sperm in semen
  (azoospermia caused by tubal obstruction or testes not producing)
- low sperm count (commonest cause)
  (oligospermia defined as < 20 000 000 sperm/mL)
- poor sperm motility
  (asthenospermia means that sperm cannot reach or penetrate an ovum)
- abnormal sperm morphology
  (teratospermia; abnormally shaped sperm reduce penetration ability).

It is not unusual for several abnormalities to coexist.

Conservative approach for subfertility

- Cease smoking tobacco
- Have more frequent intercourse
- Avoid hot baths/saunas
- Wear loose fitting underwear
- Avoid contact with pesticides (Hirsh 2003).

Treatment options

- **Drug treatments** are unlikely to improve sperm quality or motility.
- **Gonadotrophin** can help produce more sperm for those men with a deficiency of this hormone but fertility rates *are not* increased.
- **Artificial insemination** with partner's semen: *sperm is washed and concentrated (density gradient technique) and directly inserted into the uterus.*
- **In vitro fertilisation and embryo transfer (IVF–ET):** *strong sperm are selected and put in contact with the ovum in a 'test tube'. There is a 90% success rate. Failure to fertilise is indicative of sperm failure (motility, penetration of ovum).*
- **Gamete intrafallopian transfer (GIFT):** *placing sperm directly into the fallopian tube has a better chance of fertilising an ovum than the IVF–ET method.*

- **Pronuclear stage transfer (PROST):** *the IVF–ET method precedes placement of fertilised ovum into the fallopian tube.*

N. B. The women must have a general anaesthetic for egg donation and implantation just days apart.

- **Intra-cytoplasmic sperm injection (ICSI):** *for men with no sperm in their ejaculate modern technology makes it possible to fertilise an ovum from a single sperm microsurgically aspirated from the epididymis or testes. Assisted fertilisation occurs by IVT-ET.*
- **Donor insemination (anonymous or traceable):** *where there are barriers such as cost, a limitation on couples' time, frustration with timing optimal fertilisation (ovulation), complexity of the procedure and severe male infertility, the insemination with donor sperm (that has been screened for genetic problems and diseases) is a preferable option for many infertile couples.*

Role of the specialist nurse

Fertility clinics and specially trained nurse counsellors should be involved with couples from the diagnostic stage through to preferred treatment, if desired. This continuity of care is important because there is a great potential for infertility within couples to place substantial stress on their relationship and prospect of life together. Men need to be encouraged to attend the initial consultation and supported throughout in the knowledge that infertility can be a substantial threat to a male's masculine identity.

SEXUALLY TRANSMITTED INFECTIONS

Important note: Many users of this book will have been aware of resources available from the Medical Society for the Study of Venereal Diseases (MSSVD) and the Association for Genito Urinary Medicine (AGUM). The websites of these organisations have been closed because the British Association for Sexual Health and HIV (BASHH) was formed in 2003 from the merger of MSSVD and AGUM. The British Association for Sexual Health website is http://www.bashh.org/. To access AGUM resources and guidelines use http://omni.ac.uk/sitemap/ and search box for AGUM.

The terms sexually transmitted infection (STI) and sexually transmitted disease (STD) refer to any infection that can be spread through sexual activity. The United States has an epidemic of STIs with approximately 12 million new cases annually, of which 3 million occur in teenagers. England is also in the midst of a sexual health crisis with the incidence of gonorrhoea almost doubling between 1996 and 2001 and a rise in the number of cases of syphilis by 500% over the same period. In Australia the rate of gonorrhoea diagnosis increased from 23 per 100 000 in 1996 to 30 per 100 000 in 2000. The rate of chlamydia diagnosis has doubled in the same period. In the Netherlands there has been a doubling of cases of gonorrhoea among young heterosexual men and women in Amsterdam. These trends strongly suggest that the message about safer sex is being ignored by many young people. Concerns are being raised over a new generation of young gay men who appear to be ignoring messages about safer sex (Dodds et al 2000).

Groups at risk

Heterosexual men and men who have sex with men are at risk of acquiring STIs if they do not practise safe sex. Although a condom can prevent STIs the device does not protect against all STIs all of the time. There is no safe sex, only safer sex.

Although STIs have a higher incidence in lower socioeconomic groups and some ethnic groups, anyone can get a STI (FitzGerald 1997).

Although STDs appear most frequently in younger adults, any sexually active person, irrespective of their age, is at risk.

Common STIs

- Human immunodeficiency virus (HIV)
- Acquired immunodeficiency syndrome (AIDS)
- Herpes (type 1 and 2)
- Genital warts
- Syphilis
- Gonorrhoea
- Chlamydia
- Trichomoniasis
- Candidiasis
- Hepatitis B.

These infections can be transmitted during coitus, anal and oral sex and occasionally by contact with the body fluids of infected persons (e.g. blood, saliva and other secretions from mucous membranes).

General symptoms in men

- Dysuria
- Urinary frequency
- Sores or blisters on the penis, pubic area
- Pain in the scrotum
- Discharge from the penis
- Men who practise anal sex can have discharge from the rectum.

As many STIs are asymptomatic, many men do not know they have the infection. Consequently, there is a high risk of the STI being passed on to their sexual partners. Some infections (e.g. syphilis) appear to resolve themselves without treatment but actually remain active and can be passed on to others as well as causing other long term health problems.

URETHRITIS (A COMMON PRESENTATION IN MEN)

Urethritis is frequently associated with dysuria, discharge and urinary frequency. The following STIs cause urethritis:

- *Chlamydia trachomatis* (the most important cause of urethritis in heterosexual men; commonly asymptomatic). **Investigation:** first catch urinary void of the day.
- *Neisseria gonorrhoea* (found especially in men having sex with men and heterosexual men with overseas sexual contact). **Investigation:** urethral swab.
- *Herpes simplex virus* (HSV) types 1 and 2 (an uncommon cause of intermittent, recurrent attack of urethritis). **Investigation:** urethral swab.

Basic assessment

The nurse should ensure the following process is completed:

- Sexual history
- Physical examination
- Microbiology
- Serology.

Management

Syndromic

In regions where there are few resources, 'syndromic management' is often the only option. Treatment decisions are based on algorithms that refine assessment findings to the most likely cause and hence suitable treatments. Whilst this approach has been effective, people with asymptomatic STIs go largely untreated.

Best practice

In addition to diagnosis and treatment (syndromic management) the nurse should ensure that management extends to include:

- Tracing sexual contacts
- Education
- Reassurance
- Follow up
- Screening for coexisting STIs.

Opportunistic screening

Although screening of the general population is one way of identifying asymptomatic men, its effectiveness and cost effectiveness are still being evaluated. The current practice is to offer men who present with signs of an STI the opportunity to be screened for coexisting infections. It is not uncommon for more than one STI to be present. For example, some HIV positive men are practising unsafe sex and as a consequence acquire gonorrhoea. These men present with symptoms of gonorrhoea and are subsequently screened for HIV. Opportunistic screening can also be offered to men's partners who may be asymptomatic for HIV.

Where should STIs be treated?

There are several options open to people who have symptoms indicative of an STI or require information on safe sex or STIs.

1. **Genitourinary medicine** (GUM) clinics have the most comprehensive service. Advantages of GUM clinics are:
   a. Clinics are open to men and women
   b. Staff are specialised in assessment, diagnosis and treatment
   c. Staff are sensitised to patients' needs

   d. Consistency in diagnosis
   e. Consistency in treatment
   f. Consistency in contact tracing of STIs.

2. **General Practitioners.** Although GPs are able to take a health
   history and carry out basic microbial tests, additional time is
   spent sending specimens to laboratories for confirmation of
   a diagnosis. Not all GPs have the time and materials to provide
   health promotion education on safer sexual practices.

3. **Family Planning Clinics** (FPCs). Whilst women utilise FPCs
   men do not use this service for information on safer sex or
   diagnosis of genitourinary symptoms. The UK has piloted the
   combining of services in the form of a one-stop-shop for young
   people and there are recommendations to expand these
   services. Australia's 'sexually transmitted infection clinics' have
   changed their title to sexual health clinics. This reflects a
   population-based approach to sexual health where STI services
   also include family planning for both sexes.

The role of the specialist nurse

Nurses who specialise in sexual health can provide sensitive, supportive and holistic care whilst carrying out patient assessments,
performing investigative procedures, informing on diagnosis, providing treatment and tailoring discharge information specifically to
the client/patient.
   A range of services are provided:

- Tracing sexual contacts
- Education
- Reassurance
- Follow up.

Nursing issues

Consider where you might find the following information:

- the most accurate and up-to-date information on STIs'
  prevalence and trends in your country/region and population
  of interest (age, gender, ethnicity).
- updating information on *treatments and treatment issues*

- the location of national and regional services (e.g. GUM clinics)
- the location of health promotion resources for you to distribute to those most in need of safer sex (e.g. men who have sex with men, younger men)
- printed resources to hand out to patients following treatment for an STI.

Sexual health history

Prerequisites to taking a sexual history

- Be aware of one's own sexual attitude and corresponding moral judgements.
- Avoid making your judgements evident through discourse, facial expressions and body language as this may cause men to withdraw from the interview or deter them from seeking assistance or information in the future.
- Develop empathy for the patients through an understanding the psychosocial factors that influence the sexual health status of individuals and groups.
- Develop an ability to identify men most at risk of STIs without making assumptions about lifestyle and social class.
- Develop a repertoire of interview questions that improves the accuracy of data collection (last sexual contact, number of male and female partners over a specified period.

Structuring a sexual health history

- Begin with an explanation of why a history is needed.
- Acknowledge the personal and sensitive nature of the information required.
- State your role/organisation's policy in maintaining confidentiality.
- Make time to develop rapport with the man by linking your questions to what you know of his public life (this improves the rate of follow-up and options for more intense education).
- Structure a set of questions leaving time for explorative questioning.

- Proceed within professional boundaries and observe legal tenets (e.g. do not attempt to coerce the patient into consenting to treatment options; aim for a fully informed decision).
- Use language appropriate to the man's age, ethnicity and his likely cognition of concepts.
- Demonstrate interest in what the man is saying.
- Listen carefully for clues about lifestyle and barriers to his full disclosure of facts.
- Be cognisant of non-verbal cues that may indicate that a sensitive point is being raised (e.g. is sexual abuse a possibility?).
- Clarify key points with the man just prior to documenting in the case notes.

Post treatment period

Providing information does not always lead to compliance with treatment, improved health outcomes and a prevention of reoccurrence of the problem. Therefore, nurses who are cognisant of these problems use understanding, assessment, reinforcement, critical questioning and the development of individualised strategies to optimise men's sexual health.

Post treatment approach

- Understand the potential psychological impact of the diagnosis.
- Identify the possibility of the diagnosis in the sexual partners.
- Be aware of the possible concerns over their partners' fertility.
- Provide information on safer sex.
- Assess the man's understanding of the need for safer sex.
- Assess the man's cognition of how to engage in safer sex.
- Reinforce the need for abstinence during treatment.
- Reinforce the need to avoid contact with prostitutes and multiple sexual partners.

Follow up

- Was the diagnosis confirmed?
- Was mandatory notification of health authorities required?
- Did the treatment match the diagnosis?
- Was there compliance (multidose treatments)?
- Was there compliance with abstaining from intercourse?
- Are there ongoing issues (e.g. psychological, fertility of female partner)?

- Explore underlying issues such as the possibility of sexual abuse or dysfunctional sexual relationships (e.g. coercion or male prostitution).
- Reinforce the need to avoid sexual contact with persons who have symptoms (urethral discharge, lesions, warts).
- State the need for avoiding oral-genital contact (e.g. persons having oral 'cold sores').
- Reinforce the fact that not all persons with STIs have symptoms, therefore safer sex precautions are required.
- Assess the need for regular check-ups based on sexual history/risk status.
- Explore issues with sexual partners (the partner may have assumed the man was monogamous).
- Explore issues associated with seemingly heterosexual males having sex with men.
- Assess the extent to which the patient/client has presented the facts to his partner.
- Develop strategies to encourage the man to be transparent when communicating with partner(s).

If initial treatment fails:
- Check compliance.
- Ask the patient if he has been vomiting.
- Assess sexual activity since treatment.
- Consider the possibility of re-infection.
- Check that partners were treated.
- Invite partner for reassessment.

Key points

- Although STIs have a higher incidence in lower socioeconomic groups and some ethnic groups, anyone can get an STI (FitzGerald 1997).
- It is not uncommon for more than one STI to be present.
- If a man presents with symptoms indicative of an STI he should be offered the opportunity to be screened for coexisting STIs.
- Whilst information about STIs and safer sex has been well publicised, a stigma still accompanies this diagnosis.

> **Key points—cont'd**
>
> - As STIs are a sensitive social issue it is paramount that care be given by specialist nurses who are informed on how best to manage the issues and effect treatments.
> - An increase in STIs in the younger age group and in the populations in general (USA, UK, Australia, Netherlands, South East Asia) requires additional efforts and new strategies to promote safer sex.

BACTERIAL STIs

Chlamydia

Chlamydia trachomatis is the most commonly diagnosed bacterial STI in the developed world and is curable. However, as chlamydia is usually asymptomatic many cases go untreated. Chlamydia is the leading cause of pelvic inflammatory disease (Gilson & Mindel 2001). Complications include ectopic pregnancies and female infertility (Andersen et al 1998).

In men this infection causes:

- Urethritis
- Epididymo-orchitis
- Prostatitis.

Although opportunistic screening has been used, strategies for widespread screening of those at risk continue to be evaluated (Oakeshott et al 1998, Pimenta et al 2000). Male partners are less likely to present for testing because it involves a urethral swab. Andersen et al (1998) suggest that detection rates among men could be improved using home urine samples sent directly to the laboratory, as these are non-invasive and easier to collect.

Epidemiology

In the UK, between 1996 and 1999, clinics dealing with genitourinary medicine recorded a 61% increase in their case management of chlamydia (Gilson & Mindel 2001, p. 1160). In Australia this STI is the third most common notifiable infectious disease.

Symptoms

Up to 70% of women have no symptoms (Oakeshott 1997) and as such may not know that they are carriers, yet the problem can have profound effects on their fertility.
For men there can be:

* Abnormal discharge from the penis, or the anus (women have vaginal or urethral discharge)
* Inflammation around the genital area
* Pain or stinging when you pass urine
* Need to pass urine more often.

Diagnosis

Although there is no 'gold standard' for chlamydia testing, amplification assays have a sensitivity of at least 90% compared with 60–70% for culture and 60% for antigen assays (Gilson & Mindel 2001, p. 1160). Although urine samples are more time-consuming to process, the sensitivity of nucleic acid amplification tests in urine samples is high and may be higher than in urethral swabs, because of the limitations on obtaining an adequate urethral sample. Conversely, the sensitivity of a vaginal swab is higher than that of urine testing (Gilson & Mindel 2001, p. 1160).

Treatment

Although a single dose of azithromycin 1 g is more costly than the 7 day course of doxycycline, the former does not have problems associated with compliance. Despite this, the cure rate with doxycycline is 95% (Gilson & Mindel 2001, p. 1161). For cases where compliance is uncertain, a single dose of treatment may be more appropriate.

Neisseria gonorrhoea

Rates of gonorrhoea vary between developed and developing countries with the highest rates in South and South East Asia, sub Saharan Africa and Latin America (ACSHP 2001). Gonorrhoea commonly infects the male urethra. If left untreated the infection can spread to the testicles. Oral and anal infections may also occur (anal type often asymptomatic, oral often results in sore throat).

Clinical signs (men)

Gonorrhoea has similar symptoms, signs and sequelae to chlamydial infection, although symptomatic disease may be more common.

- Dysuria
- Discharge (white–yellow) from the penis (80% of cases)
- Testicular swelling and pain (advanced infection)
- Rectal infection in homosexual men may cause anal discharge (12%)
- Asymptomatic (10% of cases)
- Pharyngeal infection asymptomatic (>90%) (AGUM 2004).

Diagnosis

Specimens are collected from the urethra, rectum or oropharyngeal site, as indicated by the type of sexual activity. Microscope examination of urethral discharge and scrapings and culture (sensitivity 95%) are performed routinely. Checks for other STIs are made if the patient consents. Whilst the polymerase chain reaction (PCR) test has a high sensitivity rate relative to other methods (e.g. culture), the PCR test does not provide information about antibiotic sensitivity.

Treatment

Even when strains of gonorrhoea are sensitive to penicillin, the drug on its own is not sufficient to cure pharyngeal and anorectal infections. Therefore, for men having sex with men, ceftriaxone or ciprofloxacin is required.

Management

- Referral to GUM clinics is advised.
- This STI is a notifiable disease.
- Long term implications of uncontrolled infection need emphasising (e.g. women and sterility).
- Men and partners should be advised to abstain from sex until after treatment and follow-up.

Nursing issues

Patients should be asked if they have been travelling overseas (new strains, resistant to penicillin and other antibiotics, may have caused the infection).

Men should be told that if they have had unprotected sex, their female partners are likely to be infected even though the women may have no symptoms.

Single dose treatments are recommended, as there is generally poor compliance with multi dose regimes.

Syphilis

Syphilis is a bacterial infection caused by the spirochaete *Treponema pallidum*. The infection is primarily transmitted by sexual acts (referred to as acquired) although pregnant women can pass the infection on to their fetus via the placenta (referred to as congenital). Syphilis is not uncommon (35 600 cases in the USA in 1999). Penicillin remains the drug of choice in the treatment of syphilis and the disease is currently curable, although some strains are becoming increasingly resistant to antibiotics.

How is syphilis acquired?

Acquired infection can occur by direct contact with exudates from any skin lesion and secretions from mucous membranes during sexual contact. Transmission of the organism can occur through vaginal, anal or oral sex. The infection is commonest among men who have sex with men.

Clinical signs

Primary stage

The time between infection with syphilis and the commencement of the first signs can range from 10 to 90 days. Sores are classically single, indurated and painless with serous exudate, occurring at the site of initial invasion. Sores (chancres) normally appear on genitals, anus or in the rectum (can occur on lips and mouth). The chancre is normally firm, round, small and painless. The chancre lasts approximately 3–6 weeks and will heal without treatment.

Secondary stage

If treatment is not given the infection progresses to the secondary stage when one or more areas of skin break into a rash (rough reddish brown spots). The rash can cover the entire body including the soles of the feet and palms of the hand. This rash also disappears without treatment.

Late (tertiary) stage

The latent (hidden) stage of syphilis begins when the secondary signs disappear. Damage to the brain (dementia), heart (aortic valvular problems), large blood vessels, liver, eyes (poor vision/blindness) and nervous tissue (problems with muscle coordination) occurs in this stage of the disease.

Key points

- The use of barriers to protect against AIDS also reduces the risk of sexually transmitting syphilis but does not eliminate the risk.
- Exudates from ano-genital ulceration increase the risk of transmission of HIV infection.
- There is growing evidence to show that the risk of HIV infections increases 5–10 fold if sex involves a partner who has syphilis.

Diagnosis

Dark field microscopy is used to examine material taken from infectious sores. Syphilis antibodies are detected in infected patients' blood. However, these antibodies can remain for months even after the disease has been successfully treated. Patients presenting with late stage syphilis should be offered HIV testing.

Treatment

- The treatment of choice for early and late stage syphilis is penicillin. Patients allergic to penicillin can be treated with doxycycline.
- Patients should be advised to avoid sexual contact of any sort until treatment has been given and lesions have healed.
- Sexual partners and contacts of patients should be offered screening tests for all STIs.

Nursing issues

Health professionals may acquire the infection through contact with the patient's open lesions and barrier precautions should be taken when there is a risk of contact with a patient's blood and body fluids.

A strong index of suspicion of syphilis should be maintained in any man presenting with ano-genital lesions.

Initial sores or ulcers are painless and may spontaneously disappear without treatment, and because of this many infected men may not seek help.

Use of the latex condom does not provide complete protection against syphilis because all syphilitic sores on genital and other areas may not be covered.

Long term follow-up is required following treatment of syphilis.

If follow-up and safe sex practices are, in the judgement of the health professional, unlikely to be assured, treatment should be offered to the patient without waiting for the laboratory results.

Syphilis remains a notifiable disease in most states and provinces in most Western countries.

Trichomoniasis

Trichomonas vaginalis is a flagellated protozoan bacterium. The infection is almost exclusively sexually transmitted and is the most treatable STI. In women, this can cause infection in the vagina, urethra, and paraurethral glands. In men, infection is usually of the urethra. Prevalence is highest in those aged 20–45 years.

Symptoms

Approximately 15–50% of men are asymptomatic. Symptoms include:

- Urethral discharge, small to moderate amounts (50–60% of men)
- Dysuria
- Urinary frequency (rare)
- Urethral irritation (rare).

Diagnosis

Diagnosis is difficult, since the symptoms of **trichomoniasis** mimic those of other STDs and detection methods lack precision. Urethral culture or culture of first void urine will diagnose 60–80% of infected men. Sampling both sites will increase the diagnostic rate. Direct observation by wet mount slides or staining will only diagnose about 30% of infected men (Prodigy 2002). Polymerase chain reaction based tests, recently developed, have specificities approaching 100% (AGUM 2001).

Treatment

Give metronidazole (2 g orally, as a single dose *or* 400–500 mg twice daily for 5–7 days) as recommended by the Association of Genito Urinary Medicine (AGUM 2001). Oral metronidazole achieves a cure in 95% of cases. Sexual partners should be treated simultaneously, with abstinence from sexual contact until treatment is completed. Metronidazole resistance is on the rise, outlining the need for research into alternative antibiotics (Petrin et al 1998). Screening for coexisting STIs is recommended.

VIRAL STIs
Genital herpes (herpes simplex virus)

Epidemiology

Genital herpes (GH) is an incurable sexually transmitted infection caused by the cold sore virus. The herpes simplex virus is typed as HSV1 (usual cause of oro-labial herpes) or HSV2. Most people have an HSV – 70% facially and 10% genitally in the UK. Gilson & Mindel (2001, p. 1160) report that in 1999, in the UK, 17 456 people were diagnosed with a 'first episode' genital herpes and 14 329 with a 'recurrent episode'. Although comparable data is not available from the USA, an estimated 500 000 Americans visited the doctor for this problem in the same period. Three quarters of people with HSV don't know they have it: 1 in 4 will have no symptoms; 2 in 4 will have only mild symptoms and are unlikely to be diagnosed; 1 in 4 will have more noticeable symptoms and will be diagnosed (www.herpes.org.uk).

Risk factors (Herpes simplex type 2)

- Increasing age (acquisition most common age 15–40 years)
- Females have a higher incidence than males
- Risk increases with number of sexual partners
- Earlier age of first intercourse
- Increased number of sexual partners
- History of other STI
- Lower level of education
- Involvement with sex industry (Gilson & Mindel 2001, p. 1161)
- Female to male infection rates are less than 5% per year.

Diagnosis

Diagnosis is by clinical examination to be confirmed by culture. Successful culturing depends on:

- Using swabs taken directly from the base of the lesion
- Rapid transport of specimen to laboratory
- Maintaining the cold chain (4°C)
- Avoiding freeze–thaw cycles.

Most commercial tests for HSV antibodies are not type specific. Serological evaluation of GH requires access to HSV1 and HSV2 type assay tests. Type-specific immune responses can take 8–12 weeks to develop following the primary infection. Patients with genital herpes should be screened for other STIs, especially chlamydia.

Treatment

As many infections are mild treatment may be restricted to symptomatic relief:

- Saline bathing
- Analgesia
- Topical anaesthetic agents.

Severe infection may require antiviral medications. Oral antiviral drugs are indicated in the first 5 days of symptoms (e.g. 200 mg five times daily for five days). Aciclovir, valaciclovir and famciclovir all reduce pain, duration of symptoms and viral shedding (Oakeshott & Hay 2002). Combining oral and tropical treatment is of no benefit.

Men should receive counselling aimed at recognising that:

- a G H diagnosis often causes considerable emotional distress
- GH is common and relatively harmless (even to pregnant women)
- less than 50% have recurrent attacks (recurrence not due to reinfection)
- rate of recurrent attacks decreases with time
- recurrent episodes are often self limiting and accompanied by milder symptoms (8–10 days duration)
- Increase in life stress is not a proven trigger to recurrence
- There is a Herpes Viruses Association helpline (www.herpes.org.uk)

Counselling points require reiteration by leaflets, and men who do not adjust to diagnosis after one year should be considered for more intensive counselling.

Measures to reduce cross infection

- Contact tracing should take place.
- Partner(s) should be made aware of the diagnosis.
- Abstain from sexual intercourse whilst sores are active.
- Avoid sexual intercourse if symptoms are developing.
- The prodromal phase is accompanied by itching, tingling or numbness at site.
- Patients should be advised on the consistent use of condoms (preventing viral shedding even when asymptomatic).
- The efficacy of condoms to prevent sexual transmission is not fully evaluated.

Symptoms

- Many herpes infections are asymptomatic.
- Type 1 causes facial cold sores.
- HSV1 and 2 are the commonest causes of genital ulceration (Gilson & Mindel 2001).
- Inguinal lymphadenopathy is evident in severe cases.

Genital warts

Genital warts are caused by the human papillomavirus (HPV) and are *the most common symptomatic STI*. Infection with one of the 30 HPV types that infect genital epithelium is very common. Most infections are asymptomatic with the most usual manifestation being genital warts (most commonly types 6 and 11). The warts are nearly always transmitted by sexual contact with self-inoculation from hand to genitals being rare. The incubation period varies from 2 weeks to 8 months. Infection with 'oncogenic' strains of HPV has been shown to be a major risk factor for developing ano-genital cancers and cervical cancer (Bowden et al 2002). Condoms reduce but do not eliminate the risk of HPV cross infection.

Diagnosis

- Diagnosis of genital warts is almost always clinical.
- The role of HPV detection in general practice has not been defined.
- The smear and single HPV typing assay are available to detect most HPV types for women.

Treatment

- Cryotherapy
- Cautery/laser ablation
- Podophyllin paint (0.5%) applied twice daily for 3 consecutive days
- Trichloroacetic acid
- Vaccines remain in the developmental stage.

Hepatitis A, B and C

Men with this diagnosis should be told not to donate blood, semen or organs and should be given advice on the routes of transmission of these viruses. Hepatitis A, B and C are notifiable diseases. It is recommended that men presenting to sexual health clinics with a diagnosis of hepatitis be screened for other STIs (AGUM 2002).

Hepatitis A (incubation 15–45 days)

Hepatitis A is caused by a picorna (RNA) virus, is associated with poor sanitation and has a mortality of approximately 0.02%. Outbreaks have been reported in gay men, linked to oral-anal sex or digital-rectal contact. Vaccination of gay men is recommended in outbreak areas. Men who have multiple sexual contacts or anonymous partners are also at risk. However, several studies have shown similar prevalence between gay and heterosexual men, suggesting that most gay men are not at increased risk (AGUM 2002). Therefore, universal vaccination for this group is not recommended. Young people embarking on overseas travel to developing countries should be informed of routes of transmission and alerted to the dangers of coming into contact with sex traders. Contact sexual partners and notify public health authorities of household contacts because of possible food and water contamination.

Hepatitis B (incubation 40–160 days)

Hepatitis B is caused by a hepanda (DNA) virus, is endemic worldwide and has a mortality rate of <1% of acute cases. Aside from blood contact through skin penetration by any needle (tattoo, acupuncture, medical), the virus can be transmitted through sexual contact, oral-anal sex, rimming and coitus. Hepatitis is a notifiable disease and contact tracing should include any sexual contact (vaginal, oral or anal) or needle sharing partners (AGUM 2002).

Screening
Screening for hepatitis B should be offered to asymptomatic gay men, sex workers (male and female), sexual assault victims, intravenous drug users and sexual partners of hepatitis B positive patients or patients in other high-risk groups. Screening often takes place in countries where the infection is common, e.g. in Western Europe, North America and Australasia (AGUM 2002).

Hepatitis C (4–20 weeks)

Hepatatis C is caused by the flaviviridae family (RNA) virus. Sexual transmission occurs at a relatively low rate (0.2–2%/year of relationship, or 2–11% of spouses in long term relationship). It is estimated 2% of gay men attending GUM clinics carry hepatitis C and the rate increases if the patient is infected with HIV (AGUM 2002). Although the mortality rate is <1%, approximately 20–30% of chronic carriers develop severe liver disease up to 14–20 years after the initial infection.

Human immunodeficiency virus

While all nurses are aware of the occupational risks of acquiring HIV, most men need some form of clarification on the modes of transmission and implications for their partner and donor activities. Human immunodeficiency virus (HIV) causes acquired immune deficiency syndrome (AIDS). HIV destroys the body's ability to fight infection by attacking the immune system. This results in infected individuals becoming susceptible to opportunistic infections (e.g. tuberculosis, gonorrhoea). There are two types HIV-1 and HIV-2; both have the same means of transmission.

Modes of transmission

- Sexual (vaginal, oral or anal)
- Bloodborne transmission (sharing needles or syringes)
- Blood products (haemophiliacs affected)
- Pregnant women infecting fetus (vertical transmission).

Since 1992 all US blood donations have been screened for HIV-1 and HIV-2. The risk of transmitting HIV through open mouth kiss is rated at being very low because of the unlikelihood of blood contact. Transmission by human bites is also rare.

Nurses are often in a position to clarify modes of transmission for teenagers who are openly questioning variances in sexual activity. Many teenagers consider fellatio to be a safe means of having a sexual experience. Fellatio refers to oral contact with the penis. Cunnilingus refers to oral vaginal contact. However, over 41% of 15–17 year olds surveyed by questionnaire (USA) believed that HIV could not be contracted through fellatio or were unsure (Centre for Disease Control 2000). Oral and anal sex are not considered safe modes of sexual contact.

Infection rates

Since AIDS notification began (1982) there have been 54 261 cases in the UK. In 2000 there were 23 000 with a projected figure of 34 000 by 2005. Whilst gay and bisexual men remain the biggest risk group those in heterosexual relationships continue to be the largest group with HIV infection. This phenomenon is attributed to people coming to work and live in the UK from areas where HIV is most prevalent. It is estimated that 90% of new diagnoses (n=4300 cases) in 2002 could be attributed to heterosexuals who had become infected in sub-Saharan Africa (most often men). It is estimated that 800 000–900 000 people currently living in the USA have HIV and that 40 000 cases will occur every year. 70% of new infections occur in men. 42% of infections occur in men who have sex with men. This is followed by 33% among heterosexual relationships and 25%

in intravenous drug users (USA figures). Despite being aware of their HIV infection, a substantial number of homosexual men or bisexual men attending GUM clinics in the UK continue to practise unsafe sex (Dodds et al 2000).

Preventing transmission

The surest way of avoiding HIV or any STI is to:

- abstain from oral, anal and vaginal intercourse
- maintain a long term mutually monogamous relationship.

For condoms to reduce the risk of HIV transmission they must be used consistently and correctly. Condoms provide a high degree of protection against HIV; however, there is a 2% risk of breakage (half of the breakages estimated to be occurring prior to ejaculation). Although it has been observed that uncircumcised men have a high risk of contracting HIV, there is insufficient evidence to recommend circumcision as a means of reducing the risk of transmitting HIV.

Attitudes of healthcare workers

The following statement is designed to diminish apprehension among health and social workers concerning contact with HIV positive men. Healthcare workers have a low but measurable risk of HIV infection after accidental exposure to infected blood or body fluids. Based on over 3000 incidents, the average risk of HIV infection after a single percutaneous exposure is 0.3% (95% confidence interval 0.18%–0.46%). Contamination of mucous membranes and non-intact skin carries an even lower risk, while conjunctival contamination with blood carries a slightly higher risk. As a result HIV attributable to occupational exposure is uncommon: only 92 cases have been reported worldwide (Eastbrook & Ippolito 1997). The use of prophylactic antiretroviral agents after accidental exposure has been shown to reduce the incidence of seroconversion. The UK Department of Health recommends that healthcare workers intending to work or do part of their training overseas take a starter pack of HIV post-exposure prophylaxis (Tilzet & Banatvala 2002).

Disclosure of HIV status

In a landmark case in Australian law a woman has successfully sued two GPs for their failure to ensure that she was informed of her husband's HIV positive status. She and her husband from

Ghana were tested prior to marriage but her husband forged documents in order to convince his wife that he had a negative result.

Transmission of HIV from a health worker to a patient has never been recorded in the UK. Consequently, patients will not always be told that their carer is infected with HIV. The UK government's new sexual health strategy aims to lower HIV infections by 25%.

Screening issues

Despite official guidelines, few UK hospitals offered HIV testing as part of routine antenatal screening. Consequently, most maternal infections go undetected. Routine serological testing of GUM patients in the UK does not include screening for HIV and hepatitis C. The UK national sexual health strategy states that 40% of new patients will be screened for HIV by 2004 and 60% by 2007. The UK is considering testing migrants and asylum seekers for HIV at the point of entry. Screening for coexisting disease among HIV positive persons is highly recommended. In the USA there is concern over the 10–15 million Americans infected with tuberculosis (TB). The risk of contracting TB is far greater for those who are infected with HIV. About 25% of those infected with HIV in the USA are also infected with hepatitis C.

HIV assessment and counselling

The importance of taking an accurate sexual health history and injecting drug risk history for the man and his partner(s) cannot be overstated. The assessment needs to be conducted in a sensitive manner because poor communication will result in the man withholding information or withdrawing from the interview, making any assessment meaningless.

HIV testing

Men may present for testing for a wide range of reasons (anxiety, symptoms). For those identified as being in a high-risk group, testing should be offered and a pre-test discussion should take place on the basis of informed consent. A pre-test discussion for all men should include:

- HIV status of regular partner
- Knowing if the partner is aware of the request for the test
- Giving information concerning the HIV antibody test

- What seroconversion means
- The difference between AIDS and HIV
- The significance of the last possible exposure (12 week window period)
- Medical advantages of knowing the HIV status sooner rather than later
- How the results of the tests are obtained (via counsellor, GP or self-collection)
- Confidentiality
- Counselling available for those who are negative and positive
- Possible psychological reaction to a positive and negative test result
- Responsibility for partner notification and likely issues
- Treatment options
- An assessment of the need for more time/information to decide (Chippindale & French 2001).

Treatment

The mortality rates attributable to HIV-1 infection has declined remarkably in the UK since the introduction of antiviral drugs in 1996. New highly active antiretroviral therapies (HAART), also know as drug cocktails, have been responsible for a reduction in AIDS related deaths. However, the transmission of drug resistant HIV-1 in the UK seems to be increasing. The prevalence of transmitted HIV drug resistance in the UK exceeded 20% in 2000. Given the slower development of AIDS from HIV-2, and limited numbers of those infected, little is known about the best approach to treating HIV-2.

VASECTOMY

Vasectomy is one of the most common operations with almost 100 million men worldwide having used this method of family planning (Weiske 2001). Vasectomy provides a high level of contraception with minimal complications in most men (Preston 2000).

Methods of vas deferens occlusion

- Ligation and excision of vas deferens
- Cautery and clipping of vas deferens
- Cautery and fascial interposition (abdominal end of vas deferens).

Figure 5.1 outlines the structures within the scrotal sac and can be used to identify the vas deferens for men having the procedure. As part of the preoperative preparation the nurse should ensure that men having the procedure understand that the volume of their ejaculate will remain approximately the same. Although the ligation of the vas deferens is intended to stop all sperm leaving the testes, the total volume of sperm is very small. The obstructed sperm are absorbed by the body. Almost 60% of the volume of semen is produced by the seminal glands and the remainder by the prostate. These structures lie beyond the point of the vasectomy and so ejaculate is normal in consistency and volume.

There is no widely accepted method of vas occlusion. Figure 5.2 shows one method of ligating the vas deferens.

Effectiveness of contraception

A study of 16 796 men undergoing a vasectomy found 69 men with sperm in all semen samples taken after the procedure and 3 men became fathers as a result of not complying with the request for follow-up evaluation of their semen (Preston 2000). The most

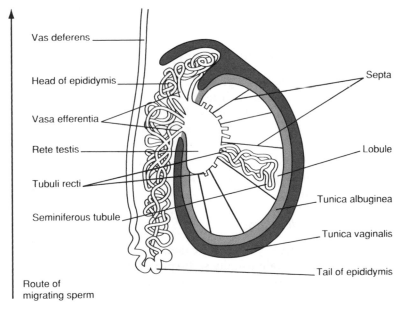

Figure 5.1   Anatomy of testes.

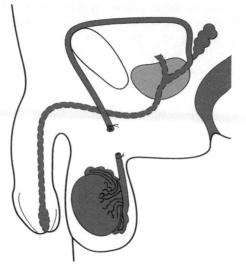

Figure 5.2   Vasectomy.

frequent cause of undesired pregnancy following vasectomy is a failure by the male to wait until azoospermia is confirmed before having intercourse. Spontaneous micro-recanalisation of the vas is a rare event (Weiske 2001).

Preoperative counselling and consent

- Both partners should be present at the decision making point.
- Permanency of the procedure must be emphasised.
- Probability of failure should be discussed.
- Social and economic implications of future pregnancy should be discussed.
- It may take months for azoospermia to occur.
- Paternity (although very rare) can occur at any time as a result of recanalisation.

Instruction on discharge

- Vasectomy is usually uncomplicated.
- Discomfort and pain usually settle promptly.
- A few patients experience local bleeding and scrotal haematoma.
- Contraception should be used until azoospermia is confirmed.

Follow up

Vasectomy is not 100% effective in preventing conception. Sperm may remain viable and motile for some time after the procedure. Post vasectomy semen analysis always consists of sedimented ejaculate. However, a variety of recommendations exist in relation to the timing of this analysis. Data in the literature range from 1–3 follow-ups, at intervals between 6 weeks and 1 year. Guidelines suggest 6 weeks, 12 weeks and 6 months (Weiske 2001).

Vasectomy reversal

Reversal of vasectomy is possible although 95% of men never request it. Men desiring reversal usually have separated from their spouse/partner and wish to have a child with another woman. Pregnancy rates achieved from reversals range from 40–75%.

ANDROGEN DEFICIENCY

Androgen deficiency (AD) affects approximately 1 : 200 men. The deficiency classically occurs due to testicular dysfunction that directly reduces testosterone output (primary hypogonadism) or hypothalamic–pituitary dysfunction that reduces pituitary luteinising hormone (LH) secretion (secondary hypogonadism). AD can be congenital or acquired. A history of orchitis, testicular trauma or other pathology may contribute to hypotestosteronaemia (Conway et al 2000, Gould 2000).

Symptoms of profound hypotestosteronaemia

- Bone loss
- Osteoporosis.

Diagnosis

Diagnosis of AD involves evaluation of testicular function through:

- History of puberty
- History of fertility (decrease in spermatogenesis)
- Changes in sexual function
- Known testicular pathology
- Testicular volume (orchidometry)
- General musculature

- Body hair growth
- Signs of gynaecomastia
- Drug use
- Occupation
- Serum testosterone and luteinising hormone (LH), follicle stimulating hormone (FSH) (Conway et al 2000).

Classical androgen deficiency is easily diagnosed. Less severe deficiency is more difficult to diagnose due to its variable clinical features and can easily be missed, denying men simple and effective medical treatment (Conway et al 2000, Andrology Australia 2003).

Androgen replacement therapy (ART)

Testosterone and not synthetic agents are recommended for the treatment of AD. ART should be initiated with intramuscular injections of testosterone esters, 250 mg every 2 weeks (ESA 1999, 2000, Conway 2000).

Androgen therapy is not recommended for:

- Professional athletes who wish to compete (disqualification)
- Older men who do not have androgen deficiency
- Male infertility.

Androgen therapy is contraindicated for:

- Men with prostate cancer
- Breast cancer.

ERECTILE DYSFUNCTION (IMPOTENCE)

Erectile dysfunction (ED) can be defined as the consistent inability to achieve or maintain an erection for the purpose of satisfactory sexual performance. An estimated 30 million men in the United States are affected by ED with less than 10% of these men seeking treatment (Charatan 1998). Impotence is defined as the persistent failure to develop erections of sufficient rigidity for penetrative sexual intercourse (Kirby 1994).

How common is ED?

Erectile dysfunction has been under-diagnosed in the past. The introduction of Viagra® (sildenafil) in 1998 in the UK resulted in an almost two fold increase in the diagnosis of erectile dysfunction between 1998 and 2000.

How does an erection occur?

Erections develop in response to a stimulus arising in the brain, where an arousal occurs in response to an image, smell or sound. Nerve impulses travel from the brain, down the spinal cord, leaving the spinal cord at its lower level and entering the penis. During sleep the brain normally stimulates an erection 3–4 times a night. Erections may also occur through local stimulation of the penis. Once stimulation occurs there is an increase in blood flow to spongy tissue shaped in the form of two tubes. Those tubes are surrounded by tough fibrous tissue that is partially elastic. Erection of the penis depends on the adequate filling of the paired corpora cavernosa with arteriole blood. The muscle cells in the spongy tissue are influenced by chemical factors that determine whether the penis is hard or soft. Erection occurs once the tonically contracted cavernosal and helicine arteries relax, increasing blood flow to the lacumar spaces and resulting in engorgement of the penis (Kirby 1994). Viagra works by stopping production of phosphodiesterase, a chemical that destroys cyclic GMO, the key chemical needed to form a normal erection. In healthy men both chemicals balance each other.

Categories of dysfunction

Erectile dysfunction has three categories with the cause occurring equally (one third) for each category.

- psychological factors
- physical factors
- both psychological and physical factors (Dinsmore & Evans 1999).

Causes of dysfunction

- Psychological
- Neurological
- Endocrinological
- Vascular (venous or arterial)
- Traumatic
- Iatrogenic (drugs and surgery) (Kirby 1994).

Risk factors for vasculogenic impotence

- Smoking tobacco
- Hypertension
- Hyperlipidaemia
- Diabetes mellitus
- Age
- Cardiovascular disease
- Hypercholesterolaemia
- The excessive use of alcohol
- Genitourinary surgery
- Psychiatric disorders
- The use of a number of prescription drugs (Kirby 1994, Kaye & Jick 2003, p. 424).

Assessment

Assessment of the patient can be carried out by any health professional competent to achieve the reasonable minimum standards for history taking and examination. The ideal service for assessing, treating and monitoring men with ED in secondary care should be multidisciplinary. The specialist nurse, appropriately trained, is ideally placed to play a key role in ensuring a continuity of care for men with ED and monitoring the effects and outcomes of treatment and may even hold agreements on prescribing rights: 'This role may amount to total patient management' (Ralph & McNicholas 2000).

Specialist nurses should refer to their governing bodies to determine their scope of and standards of practice. For example, the Nurses Board of New South Wales (http://www.nursesreg.nsw. gov.au/bounds/guidelin.htm); the Australian Nursing Council (http://www.anc.org.au/competencystandards.htm); the UK Central Council for Nursing, Midwifery and Health Visiting; *The Scope of Professional Practice* (UKCC 1992); the Nursing and Midwifery Council (http://www.nmc-uk.org/cms/content/home/search. asp).

Making an assessment

Detailed personal history (the most important part of the assessment)

The focus of history taking is to determine the cause of the complaint and the expectations and motivation of the man (and his partner) for further diagnosis and treatment. A drug history is essential since many commonly used drugs have been implicated with erectile dysfunction (Kirby 1994). Treatment of ED using drugs may not be an option if they are likely to interact with the patient's medication taken for other health problems.

Mandatory items

- Blood pressure
- Urinalysis for glucose
- Examination of the genitalia (testicular size, any fibrosis in the shaft of the penis, retractability of the foreskin).

Identifying mental health problems

- Anxiety states
- Gender identity problems.

History of psychiatric illnesses

- Depressions
- Psychosis
- Body dysmorphic disorder.

Medications used in the management of these illnesses may be linked to ED. Pharmacotherapy or implantation of prostheses will fail in patients whose problem is primarily psychogenic (Kirby 1994).

Investigations or further examination

Salient investigations for the individual will be determined by the overall history given at interview and the findings of a physical examination. Investigations might include cardiovascular, neurological and endocrine systems.

Endocrine investigations

If there is a reduced sex drive blood should be sent for measurement of concentrations of:

- LH
- Prolactin – especially for reduced sex drive in young men
- Testosterone – total serum

- Sex hormone binding globulin (SHBG)
- Free androgen index (FAI) (Kirby 1994, Dinsmore & Evans 1999).

A testosterone level may be taken on the basis that a physical examination reveals hypogonadism or may more commonly be taken to reassure patients that testosterone is not implicated with their ED. A liver function test may be performed on the basis of the history revealing alcohol abuse or hepatitis. An abnormal liver function is linked with ED. A history of diabetes may be linked to renal impairment/problems indicating that a dipstick urine analysis and creatinine level test should be performed. Afro-Caribbean patients should have their haemoglobin tested to exclude the possibility of sickle cell disorder.

Other possible investigations

- Presence of nocturnal erections
- Vascular function.

Testing of nocturnal penile tumescence in hospital has been replaced by self-administered tests of nocturnal erections such as the snap gauge band and Rigiscan device. Vascular function can be assessed by Doppler colour ultrasound, response to injections, arteriography. Colour Doppler imaging after inducing maximal intra-cavernous smooth muscle relaxation using papaverine provides detailed information about the haemodynamics of the penis and is particularly useful in distinguishing between arterial insufficiency and veno-occlusive dysfunction (Kirby 1994). However, Dinsmore and Evans (1999) state that: 'surgery for venous leakage and microvascular techniques for revascularisation of the corpora are rarely done, and the results are not good.'

Medications implicated with ED

- Beta blockers (used as antihypertensives, e.g. propanolol, atenolol)
- Diuretics (thiazide, spironolactone, triamterene, acetazolamide)
- Antidepressants
- Antipsychotics
- Anticonvulsants

- Anti-Parkinson's disease drugs
- Hormonal agents
- Lipid lowering agents
- H2 antagonists.

What treatments are available?

It is important that any psychiatric problem be identified and addressed before treatment for ED is recommended or commenced. Patients should be given advice on expected treatment outcomes and a follow-up consultation should be based on goals established at the start of treatment. Patients should be advised on what to do should they experience problems with treatments or complications from treatments (Ralph & McNicholas 2000). Follow-up is also important as a means of auditing outcomes. A review between 4 and 6 weeks allows for a change in or cessation of treatment. However, a longer term follow-up is advised for men using injections as there is a possibility of penile fibrosis developing.

Injectable preparations

Prostaglandin can be directly injected by the intracavernosal route just prior to coitus. Men and their partners need to assess the discomfort, the need for spontaneity of coitus and ease of use when choosing injectable treatments as this affects compliance.

Side effects

- Penile fibrosis from multiple injection sites or reactions to injectables
- Bruising
- Pain
- Priapism (an erection lasting longer than 6 hours).

Alprostadil (prostaglandin E) is supplied in 5, 10 and 20 µg doses. Patients are normally commenced on low doses in clinical settings and informed that the effect is improved in the more relaxed environment of the patient's home. The lower doses are likely to be effective in counteracting the effects of neurological disease (Dinsmore & Evans 1999).

Oral medications

Sildenafil (Viagra®)

Sildenafil (Viagra®) is an important development in the treatment of erectile dysfunction. It enhances the vasodilation effect of endogenous nitric acid leading to the release of nitric oxide, an essential part of the erectile process (Dinsmore & Evans 1999). In 21 clinical trials conducted on 4000 men, sildenafil citrate was found to be effective in 70% of cases (Charatan 1998). The most effective dose appears to be 50–100 mg with minimal side effects. It has been suggested that this oral treatment may lose its effect over time. However, further research is required to establish and test this hypothesis.

Advantages
Sildenafil can be taken an hour before intercourse (Charatan 1998) and priapism has not been reported.

Disadvantages
The most common side effect is a headache. Other side effects include facial flushing, indigestion, a stuffy nose and a very small percentage of men report a blue tinge to their vision.

Contraindications
A major contraindication of this drug is ischaemic heart disease; it is also contraindicated in men treated with organic nitrates (e.g. glyceryl trinitrate) because the combined effect may cause hypotension (Charatan 1998).

Yohimbine

Yohimbine has been used for many decades but it has not been licensed and there is no long term data available on its toxicology (Dinsmore & Evans 1999). A signed consent for treatment needs to be gained where products that are unlicensed are used (e.g. papaverine, vasoactive intestinal polypeptide).

Oral administration is of yohimbine 5 mg, three times a day or 5–15 mg 1 hour before intercourse. Although there are claims that it is effective in 50% of patients, it is thought that there is a significant placebo effect.

Contraindications
Should not be used in patients with severe hypertension.

Testosterone

Testosterone may be given orally although it is usually given as an intramuscular depot injection at periods of 3–4 weeks. Daily patches or 6-monthly implants may also be used.

Contraindications

Patients with suspected or confirmed carcinoma of the prostate are contraindicated. Serum levels of PSA should be checked every 6 months as an indicator of prostatic problems.

Patients with normal serum testosterone should not be given this treatment as it may exacerbate the problem by increasing sexual drive without improvements in performance.

Transurethral route

Prostaglandin

Prostaglandin (alprostadil) is given transurethrally to bring about erection of the penis. However, for those patients with an organic cause of ED outcomes vary. fewer than 65% of users achieved an erection sufficient for intercourse over a 3 month period of home therapy.

The medicated urethral system for erection (MUSE)

The MUSE system requires that prior to sex men need to urinate, insert a small applicator into their meatus, travelling an inch down the urethra, press a button that releases a tiny pellet of prostaglandin (alprostadil) and massage the penis to help dissolve the pellet. The pellets come in doses of 125, 250, 500 and 1000 µg and can produce an erection within 15 minutes. Whilst the method is easy to use, there is a relatively high incidence of penile pain associated with the application process and this may make patients reticent to continue with treatment for long periods.

Inflatable devices

Inflatable devices have come a long way since their inception in the 1970s. Men choosing a prosthesis usually have had little success with other options because they have either had pelvic surgery or have atherosclerosis. The prosthesis is coated in silicone and comes in either a two part prosthesis with a combined reservoir and pump that is situated in the scrotum or as three pieces with a pump located in the scrotum and a reservoir positioned in the lower part of the abdominal wall. With multipart prostheses the compartments are filled with saline with the pump located in a dependent position within the scrotum, and the reservoir under the rectus sheath (Kirby 1994). Insertion of the prosthesis into the corpora may be difficult in patients with a fibrotic penis, with Peyronie's plaques and after priapism. Semi-rigid devices require a circumcision.

Postoperative management

- Pain relief is essential as the procedure causes much discomfort and pain.
- Broad spectrum antibiotics are given orally for at least a week.

Vacuum devices

Vacuum devices fit over the penis and are applied manually or by an electrical motor (battery powered). The vacuum created draws venous blood into the penis. Once an erection has formed, the blood is dammed off using a rubber constriction ring. Although these devices are deemed safe, erections using the ring should not be maintained for longer than 30 minutes as a reduction in circulation will cause pain and tissue will become ischaemic. Vacuum devices are a useful alternative when injectables have failed or the man is averse to injections.

Psychosexual therapy

On the basis of evidence obtained from expert committee reports and the opinions or clinical experience of respected authorities, Ralph & McNicholas (2000) state that: 'A review of all outcome studies in psychosexual therapy published since 1970 showed successful outcomes in 50–80% of patients.' However, the success of psychosexual therapy requires the patient to be motivated to work with the therapist to identify factors that prevent normal sexual arousal. A successful outcome may also depend on the use of psychosexual therapy in conjunction with physical therapies.

What should a patient be told about treatments?

Treatments are determined by identified causes of ED and most ED has multifactorial causes (i.e. organic and psychological factors need to be treated).

When choosing treatments patients should:

- be provided with information on all suitable treatment options in a manner that is not biased by the professional's personal choice/manufacturers' unsupported claims
- be informed on the ease of use and overall costs
- be provided with information about known significant risks, at a level of knowledge and terminology congruent with the patient's cultural background and general understanding of ED, so as to facilitate a fully informed decision
- be given time to debate and evaluate the merit of options so that, in the final choice, it can be assured that the treatment is to the patient's needs and preferences and, where applicable, to those of his partner
- be made aware of the benefits of having his sexual partner present at appointments that focus on the choice of treatment
- agree on treatment goals established before treatment starts
- develop an action plan and identify a contact person (health professional who has a history of prior consultations) should complications arise from treatments or when a problem occurs with the use of treatments.

References

Andrology Australia 2003 Men's health matters: androgen deficiency. Is low testosterone putting me in the slow lane? Andrology Australia, Monash Institute of Reproduction and Development, Victoria

Association of Genitourinary Medicine (AGUM) 2001 National guidelines on the management of Trichomoniasis vaginalis. Clinical Effectiveness Group (Association of Genitourinary Medicine and Medical Society for the Study of Venereal Diseases). The AGUM website is closed. Use: http://www.bashh. org/ guidelines/2002/tv_0601.pdf

Association of Genitourinary Medicine (AGUM) 2002 National guidelines on the management of the viral hepatitides A, B and C. Clinical Effectiveness Group (Association of Genitourinary Medicine and Medical Society for the Study of Venereal Diseases). The AGUM website is closed. Use National Guideline Clearinghouse™ (NGC) 2002 National guideline on the management of the viral hepatitides A, B, and C: http://www.guidelines.gov/summary/ summary. aspx?doc_id=3454&nbr=2680&string=hepatitis

Association of Genitourinary Medicine (AGUM) 2004 National guidelines on the management of gonorrhoea in adults. Clinical Effectiveness Group (Association of Genitourinary Medicine and Medical Society for the study of Venereal Diseases). The AGUM website is closed. Use: http://www.bashh.org/ guidelines/ draft_04/draft_gonorrhoea_guideline_2004.doc

Australian College of Sexual Health Physicians (ACHSP) 2001 Clinical guidelines for the treatment of sexually transmissible infections among priority populations. ACSHP. Online. Available: http://www.acshp.org. au/sexual_health/publications/_STI_Management_Priority_poulations.pdf

Andersen B, Ostergaard L, Moller JK et al 1998 Home sampling versus conventional contact tracing for detecting *Chlamydia trachomatis* infection in male partners of infected women: randomised study. British Medical Journal 316(7128): 350–351

Bowden FJ, Tabrizi SN, Garland SM et al 2002 Sexually transmitted infections: new diagnostic approaches and treatments. Medical Journal of Australia 176 (11): 551–557

Center for Disease Control 2000 Preventing the sexual transmission of HIV, the virus that causes AIDS: what you should know about oral sex. Department of Health and Human Services, US Government

Charatan C 1998 First pill for male impotence approved in US. British Medical Journal 316(7138): 1111

Chippindale S, French L 2001 HIV counselling and the psychological management of patients with HIV or AIDS. British Medical Journal 322(7301): 1533–1535

Conway AJ, Handelsman DJ, Lording DW et al 2000 Use, misuse and abuse of androgens. The Endocrine Society of Australia consensus guidelines for androgen prescribing. Medical Journal of Australia 172(7): 220–224. [Erratum on p. 334]

Dinsmore W, Evans C 1999 ABC of sexual health: erectile dysfunction. British Medical Journal 318(7180): 387–390

Dodds JP, Nardone A, Merccey DE et al 2000 Increase in high risk sexual behaviour among homosexual men, London 1996–1998: cross sectional, questionnaire study. British Medical Journal 320(7248): 1510–1511

Eastbrook P, Ippolito G 1997 Prophylaxis after occupational exposure to HIV. British Medical Journal 315(7108): 557–558

Endocrine Society of Australia (ESA) 1999 Position statement on use and misuse of androgens. Online. Available: http://www.racp.edu.au/esa/posstat.htm

Endocrine Society of Australia (ESA) 2000 Position statement on growth hormone replacement of growth hormone deficiency in adults. Online. Available: http://www.racp.edu.au/esa/posstat.htm

FitzGerald M 1997 Gonorrhoea and ethnicity. British Medical Journal 315(7116): 1160

Gilson R, Mindel A 2001 Sexually transmitted infections. British Medical Journal 322(7295): 1160–1164

Gould DC, Petty R, Jacobs HS 2000 For and against: the male menopause–does it exist? Education and Debate. British Medical Journal 320(7238): 858

Hirsh A 2003 ABC of subfertility: male subfertility. British Medical Journal 327(7416): 669

Kaye J, Jick H 2003 Incidence of erectile dysfunction and characteristics of patients before and after the introduction of sildenafil in the United Kingdom: cross sectional study with comparison patients. British Medical Journal 326(7386): 424

Kirby RS 1994 Impotence: diagnosis and management of male erectile dysfunction. Fortnightly Review. British Medical Journal 308(6934): 957–961

Oakeshott P 1997 Vaginal discharge and sexually transmitted disease. In: McPherson A, Waller D (eds) Women's health, 4th edn. Oxford University Press, Oxford

Oakeshott P;Hay P 2002 10 minute consultation 'Genital herpes'. British Medical Journal 324(7345): 1076.

Oakeshott P, Kerry S, Hay S et al 1998 Opportunistic screening for chlamydial infection at time of cervical testing in general practice: prevalence study. British Medical Journal 316(7128): 351

Petrin D, Delgaty K, Bhatt R et al 1998 Clinical and microbiological aspects of *Trichomonas vaginalis*. Clinical Microbiology Reviews 11(2): 300–317

Pimenta J, Catchpole M, Gray M et al 2000 Screening for genital chlamydial infection. British Medical Journal, 321(7261): 629.

Preston JM 2000 Vasectomy: common medicological pitfalls. British Journal of Urology International 86(3): 339–343

Prodigy Guidance 2002 Trichomoniasis. National Health Service. Online. Available: http://www.prodigy.nhs.uk/guidance.asp?gt=Trichomoniasis

Ralph D, McNicholas 2000 UK management guidelines for erectile dysfunction. British Medical Journal 321(7259): 499–503

Tilzet AJ, Banatvala E 2002 Protection from HIV on electives: questionnaire survey of UK medical schools. British Medical Journal 325(7371): 1010–1011

Tweed MJ, Roland JM 1998 Haemochromatosis as an endocrine cause of subfertility. British Medical Journal 316(7135): 915–916

UKCC 1992 The scope of professional practice. UKCC, London

Weiske W H 2001 Vasectomy. Andrologia 33(3): 125–134

Further reading

International Journal of Impotence Research

Litwin MS, Nied RJ, Dhanani N 1998 Health-related quality of life in men with erectile dysfunction. Journal of General Internal Medicine 13(3): 159–166

Pryce A 2000 Frequent observation: sexualities, self-surveillance, confession and the construction of the active patient. Nursing Inquiry 7(2): 103–111

Pryce A 2001 Governmentality, the iconography of sexual disease and 'duties' of the STI clinic. Nursing Inquiry 8(3): 151–161

Resources

Australian Society for HIV Medicine has a number of publications to assist nurses specialising in HIV and these can be purchased online. The website is: http://www.ashm.org.au/search.php

Publications include:

HIV Management in Australasia: a guide for clinical care. This is the 4th Monograph produced by ASHM and was released in May 2003.

HIV/viral hepatitis: a guide for primary care. The guide aims to provide GPs and other interested clinicians and healthcare workers with an introduction to HIV and viral hepatitis.

Coinfection – HIV and viral hepatitis: a guide for clinical management. This is the 5th Monograph produced by ASHM and was released in April 2003.

The Australasian Contact Tracing Manual, 2nd Edition, 2002. This is an invaluable resource for all healthcare workers involved with sexual health, HIV, viral hepatitis and HIV-related tuberculosis.

A complete list of sexual health clinics in Australia and New Zealand can be accessed through the Australasian chapter of Sexual Health website: http://www.acshp.org.au/sexual_health/clinics/default.htm

EQUIP 2005 UK find your nearest registered practitioner. Sexually Transmitted Infection Clinic (Genitourinary Medicine Clinic): http://www.equip.nhs.uk/services/find.html

Alternatively, use British Association for Sexual Health and HIV: http://www.bashh.org/directory.htm

Chapter 6

Maturity

CHAPTER CONTENTS

From the age of 50 years and onward there is a substantial increase in the incidence and range of health problems for men. Conditions such as coronary artery disease and hypertension have been chosen for inclusion in this chapter because they affect a large proportion of men and, to a large extent, can be prevented by modification of lifestyle behaviours (smoking, diet, alcohol abuse). This chapter also focuses on the degenerative conditions related to declines in hormone levels as they affect strength and sexual activity as well as having psychosocial implications. The information presented here is intended to provide nurses with knowledge that can be used to dispel myths about the relationship between ageing males and their hormone levels.

TESTOSTERONE IN DECLINE

Men concerned about the ageing process are likely to ask nurses and health professionals about the effects of ageing on testosterone levels. This section provides a background briefing for nurses who want to know the ins and outs of male hormones and to dispel some of the myths for their male patients/clients. The term *androgens* denotes male sex hormones and they are based on the structure of testosterone. Testosterone is capable of creating and maintaining male sexual characteristics and fertility. The effects of testosterone on non-reproductive tissue are:

- Growth of bone
- Growth of muscle
- Promotes red blood cell production
- Affects mood state
- Mental agility.

Testosterone levels

- Peak in men between 20 and 30 years of age
- Decline naturally with age
- Have a diurnal range.

Serum testosterone

- Young men have a lower limit of 350 ng/dl.
- 40% of men > 60 years have levels < 350 ng/dl.
- By 80 years total testosterone concentrations have fallen by 75%.
- 300 ng/dl seems to be the lower level at which sexual function declines (Gould et al 2000).

Bioavailability of testosterone

An increase in sex hormone binding globulin concomitant with a reduction in total testosterone reduces the bioavailability of testosterone. Gould et al (2000) assert that concentrations of bioavailable testosterone decrease by as much as 50% in men aged 25–75 years. Obesity and excess intake of alcohol lower concentration of bioavailable testosterone.

Testosterone and sexual function

There are several fundamental points that nurses should be discussing with men who want to be informed about sexual function. Firstly, testosterone concentrations found to be critical in reducing sexual function lie below 300 ng/dL (10.4 nmol/L). Only 20% of elderly men have levels < 300 ng/dL (Weksler 1996). Despite this, Jacobs (2000) argues that circulating testosterone levels in older men are usually well above the level to maintain sexual desire. And whilst testosterone deficiency can be found for 6–45% of cases, erectile dysfunction (ED) in elderly men is most often of a non-hormonal aetiology (Gould et al 2000). Moreover, reduced sexual activity is more likely to be associated with ED than with low testosterone levels.

Secondly, the administration of testosterone may increase sexual desire but it does not improve erectile performance. This is because ED is usually a multifactorial condition with 80% of men having ED attributed to medical problems (diabetes, cardiovascular problems, neurological disorders).

Male menopause

It has been theorised that men may experience a diminution of their sex hormones and as a consequence may experience menopausal symptoms. However, male menopause is a term that is used conveniently rather than accurately because menopause refers to a winding down and cessation of the female menstrual cycle. Weksler (1996) states that the term andropause is also incorrect in the physiological sense because in contrast to women, gonadal function in men is not arrested at any age and many men retain fertility into old age.

Age related androgen deficiency (AD)

Plasma testosterone concentrations decline in men from early middle age. There is considerable variation in serum testosterone concentrations between individuals and between age groups.

Symptoms and signs

- Depressed mood
- Fatigue
- Reduced muscle mass and strength
- Demineralisation of bone
- Deposition of upper body fat
- Reduced sexual activity.

Hormone replacement therapy

Whilst there is strong evidence to show that hormone replacement therapy (HRT) can prevent some of the ills and infirmities that follow the menopause (hypo-oestrogenic symptoms) there is no conclusive evidence to show that androgen replacement therapy (ART) for men will have similar success. The evidence is suggestive that ART improves the quality of men's lives. Debate about evidence and issues surrounding ART are detailed by Gould et al (2000) along with letters of response published in the British Medical Journal.

The Endocrine Society of Australian has a position statement on the use and misuse of androgens. This statement can be accessed on the web address http://www.racp.edu.au/esa/posstat2.htm. Concerns about the safety of HRT have been raised on the basis of increasing evidence that suggests the risk of breast cancer rises in conjunction with HRT. Similar risks are possible for ART.

Androgen therapy is:
* **not recommended** for older men who do not have androgen deficiency
* **contraindicated** for men with prostate cancer.

Key points

* Androgen deficiency is an uncommon cause of erectile dysfunction.
* All men presenting with ED should be evaluated for AD.
* There is no indication for ART in male infertility.
* ART is only of value to men diagnosed with AD (hypotestosteronaemia)
* There is no convincing evidence that, where AD *is not* the diagnosis, men will benefit from ART.
* There has been no systematic research to show that HRT for men is effective in arresting or reversing symptoms of age related androgen deficiency.
* Men should be counselled about the risks, benefits and uncertainties of ART prior to commencing and stopping treatment.

MEN AND CARDIOVASCULAR DISEASE

The term cardiovascular disease is an aggregate of conditions that include:

- Coronary artery disease (CAD)
- Ischaemic heart disease (IHD)
- Hypertension.

Cardiovascular disease can lead to angina, myocardial infarction and stroke. Men develop cardiovascular disease earlier in life than women, experience more severe CAD and are more likely to die from heart disease than women. In the 35–65 age group, five times more men than women die from cardiovascular disease.

Ischaemic heart disease (IHD) is the most common cause of heart failure in men of all ages. Men with heart failure are more likely to have a habitually higher intake of alcohol and smoke cigarettes.

Primary risk factors

The primary factors for CAD include:

- Age
- Positive familial history
- Genetic and familial predisposition.

A substantial decline in the rates of IHD and CAD has been attributed to people modifying their lifestyles. This suggests that environmental factors can play a significant role in offsetting the genetic expressions for these diseases.

Modifiable risk factors

- Diabetes
- Smoking
- Sedentary lifestyle
- Central obesity
- Elevated serum low density lipoproteins (LDL)
- Low serum high density lipoproteins (HDL).

Hyperlipidaemia

For several decades there has been general consensus that high intakes of saturated fat increase plasma cholesterol levels and the risk of coronary heart disease (CHD). However, it is most likely that dietary intake and genetic variant alleles act in combination to determine an individual's susceptibility or resistance to CHD (Campos 1998). The National Service Framework (see http://www. dh.gov.uk/policyAndGuidance/HealthAndSocialCareTopics/fs/ en#5036518) suggests a cholesterol level of 5.0 mmol/L. However, 66% of men have a level above 5.0 mmol/L and the average is approximately 5.5 mmol/L.

Cigarette smoking

In general, smoking decreases the age of the time of the first CHD event by nearly one decade (Stenchever 2003). Male smokers are affected by CAD much earlier in life than women because premenopausal levels of female hormones are cardiac protective. It is estimated that about 20% of deaths from coronary heart disease in men and 17% in women are due to smoking (BHF 2003). The following points should be noted:

- Stopping smoking halves the additional risk of CHD after one year's cessation.
- Those who cease smoking for 15 years have the same risk of CHD as those who never smoked (provided all other factors are equal).
- Cessation of smoking after myocardial infarction is associated with a 50% reduction in mortality after 3–5 years (Wilson et al 2000).

Testosterone

Recent research indicates that male sex hormones, the androgens (e.g. testosterone), activate genes that are involved in the onset of CAD. However, women who have testosterone replacement do not experience similar rates of heart disease. The reason for this is that women have only one quarter of the number of androgen receptors that men have. This relatively new discovery could prompt the development of gender specific treatments.

Obesity

This is a well-established risk factor for male adult CAD. Recent research shows obesity is also associated with accelerated coronary atherosclerosis in adolescent and young adult men (McGill 2002).

Alcohol

Although moderate alcohol intake has been linked to a decrease in IHD mortality, intake of large amounts at a time may be harmful. A heavy drinking pattern (six or more drinks at a time) among working age male drinkers (25–64 years) is related to increased mortality from heart disease and cardiomyopathy (Laatikainen et al 2003).

Hypertension

High blood pressure is an important risk factor for cerebral vascular accidents (stroke) and myocardial infarction. Hypertension is often symptomless and therefore men would benefit greatly from screening for this condition. Hypertension is defined as pressure readings taken over several days and at different times that are consistently:

- 100 mmHg diastolic blood pressure (DBP) for < 65 years
- 105 mmHg diastolic blood pressure (DBP) for > 65 years.

Psychosocial factors

There is a growing body of research that implicates psychosocial well being with risk of CHD. The following factors are associated with increased risk:

- Inadequate social support (reported by 16% of men and 13% of women)
- Lack of social networks
- Employment stress (high demand combined with lack of control)
- Depression
- Personality type (A type/hostile).

CAD risk reduction

Brief behavioural counselling based on simple advice and matched to 'stage of readiness for change' is likely to be valuable in assisting those at risk of cardiovascular disease to choose a healthier lifestyle (Steptoe et al 2001). Important advice includes:

- Abstinence from smoking
- Habitual physical activity
- Avoidance of weight gain with age
- Responsible limited alcohol intake
- Reduce sodium intake (less than 2 g or 88 mmol per day)
- Diet low in saturated fatty acids and trans-fatty acids
- Diet with adequate monosaturated and polysaturated (especially omega 3) fatty acids (Lichtenstein 2003).

Hypertension

Around 40% of men have elevated blood pressures (>140/ 90 mmHg). Aside from tobacco use, this is the second most important cause of death and disability. Although the British Hypertension Society (1998) has clearly defined goals for the management of hypertension (diastolic blood pressure < 90 mmHg), approximately half of those receiving treatment do not achieve an acceptable level of control over their blood pressure. The sequelae of uncontrolled hypertension include heart disease, kidney disease and stroke.

Blood pressure thresholds

The thresholds for intervention with drug therapy are shown in Table 6.1. N. B. A threshold of 160/100 means a systolic BP of >160 mmHg or a diastolic BP of >100 mmHg. Thresholds for intervention are recorded as initial blood pressure (mmHg).

Treatment

Treatment should be based on the degree of hypertension. Use non-pharmacological measures in all hypertensive and borderline

Table 6.1   Threshold for interventions

Blood pressure	Action
<135/85	Reassess in 5 years
135/85–139/89	Reassess yearly
140/90–159/99	If there is no target organ damage or cardiovascular complications or diabetes then observe and reassess CHD risk yearly
140/90–159/99	If there is target organ damage or cardiovascular complications or diabetes then treat hypertension along with these problems
160/100–199/109	Treat hypertension even though there may be no clear evidence of target organ damage or cardiovascular complications or diabetes
>200/110	Confirm there is continuity of this pressure over 1–2 weeks then treat. However, if this pressure correlates with a hypertensive emergency or malignant hypertension, treat immediately

Adapted from British Hypertension Society Guidelines (Williams et al 2004).

hypertensive people (e.g. exercise, meditation). In patients with mild hypertension but no cardiovascular complications or target organ damage, the response to these measures should be observed during the initial 4–6 month period. When drug treatment needs to be instigated, non-pharmacological measures should be used in an effort to minimise drug dosage. In the absence of contraindications or compelling indications for other antihypertensive agents, low dose thiazide diuretics or β-blockers are preferred as first line treatment for the majority of hypertensive people. The treatment target is a systolic of 140 mmHg and a diastolic of 85 mmHg (lower for those with diabetes) (British Hypertension Society 1998).

Evaluation

All men diagnosed with hypertension should be physically examined, have a detailed health history and have the following tests as a means of identifying cause:

- Urine strip test for blood and protein
- Serum electrolytes and creatinine
- Plasma glucose
- Serum total HDL : cholesterol ratio
- 12 lead ECG (Ramsay et al 1999).

References

British Heart Foundation 2003 B3 Coronary Heart Disease Statistics Book. Online. Available: http://www.bhf.org.uk/publications/ description.asp?secondlevel=416&artID-708

British Hypertension Society 1998 Management guidelines in essential hypertension. Heart 80 (suppl 2): 21–29

Campos H 1998 Gene–diet interactions, plasma lipoproteins, and coronary heart disease: potential role of the apoAI-CIII-AIV gene cluster. Papers presented at the Australasian Clinical Nutrition Society Symposium, 2 October 1998. Australian Journal of Nutrition and Dietetics 55(4): Suppl S12–S15

Gould DC, Petty R, Jacobs HS 2000 Education and debate: the male menopause–does it exist? (the case for). British Medical Journal 320 (7238): 858

Jacobs HS 2000 Education and debate the male menopause–does it exist? (the case against). British Medical Journal 320 (7238): 858

Laatikainen T, Manninen L, Poikolainen K et al 2003. Increased mortality related to heavy alcohol intake pattern. Journal of Epidemiology and Community Health 57(5): 379–384.

Lichtenstein AH 2003 Dietary fat and cardiovascular disease risk: quality and quantity? Journal of Women's Health 12(2): 109–114

McGill HC, McMahan CA, Herderick EE et al 2002 Obesity accelerates the progression of coronary atherosclerosis in young men. Circulation 105(23): 2712–2718

Ramsay LE, Williams B, Johnston GD et al 1999 British Hypertension Society guidelines for hypertension management: summary. British Medical Journal 319(7210): 630–635

Stenchever MA 2003 Most people with CHD have conventional risk factors. ACOG Clinical Review 8(10): 13 Nov–Dec

Steptoe A, Kerry S, Rink E et al 2001 The impact of behavioural counselling on stage of change in fat intake, physical activity, and cigarette smoking in adults at increased risk of coronary heart disease. American Journal of Public Health 91(2): 265–269

Wekslar ME 1996 Book review of Carruthers M 1996 The male menopause: restoring vitality and virility. British Medical Journal 313: 1214

Wilson K, Gibson N, Willan A et al 2000 Effect of smoking cessation on mortality after myocardial infarction: meta-analysis of cohort studies. Archives of Internal Medicine 160(7): 939–944

Further reading

Brown MJ, Cruickshank JK, Dominiczak AF et al 2003 Better blood pressure control: how to combine drugs. Journal of Human Hypertension 17: 81–86. Online. Available: http://www.hyp.ac.uk/bhs/resources/ABCD.pdf

Resources

British Hypertension Society http://www.hyp.ac.uk/bhs/home.htm British Heart Foundation http://www.bhf.org.uk/

Joint British Societies Coronary Risk Prediction Chart http://www.sign.ac.uk/guidelines/fulltext/40/annex11.html

Accessed through http://www.sign.ac.uk/guidelines/fulltet/40/annex11.html *which is part of the British National Formulary* (BNF.org). *Note: The prediction chart makes it obvious that premenstrual women have hormones that are cardiac protective.*

National Service Frameworks, Department of Health, UK http://www.dh.gov.uk/PolicyAndGuidance/HealthAndSocialCareTopics/fs/en#50365

Stergiou G, Mengden T, Padfield PL et al 2004 Self monitoring of blood pressure at home. British Medical Journal 329 (7471): 870–871

Campbell NC, Murchie P 2004 Treating hypertension with guidelines in general practice. British Medical Journal 329 (7465): 523–524

Hébert K 2004 NICE sets out guidelines for hypertension. British Medical Journal 329 (7464): 475

Laurent S 2004 Guidelines from the British Hypertension Society. British Medical Journal 328 (7440): 593–594.

Williams B, Poulter NR, Brown MJ et al 2004 The BHS Guidelines. Working party guidelines for management of hypertension. Report of the Fourth Working Party of the British Hypertension Society–BHS IV. Journal of Human Hypertension 18: 139–185. Online. Available: http://www.bhsoc.org/pdfs/BHS_IV_Guidelines.pdf

A summary version of this can be had from: Williams B, Poulter NR, Brown MJ et al 2004 The BHS Guidelines Working Party. British Hypertension Society guidelines for hypertension management – BHS IV: summary. British Medical Journal 328: 634–640

Chapter 7

Sensitive issues

In any culture there are sensitive issues and often these issues have a gender base. The 5 issues selected for inclusion in this chapter represent issues that are prominent in contemporary literature and therefore highlight the need for the dissemination of knowledge, appropriate practice and the development of health promotion strategies based on systematic research. The information is presented as a background briefing with implications for practice and referral to resources.

DATE RAPE

Date rape is a controversial crime because getting sex through physical violence is clearly seen as rape by the general public, However, date rape may not involve physical violence. Other forms of coercion to obtain sex, such as the fear of violence, detention, intoxication with alcohol or a drug, and deception can all be factors relevant to whether the woman has consented. Offenders sometimes spike the drinks of victims (some of the drugs used have been put into liquid forms and dyed to make their detection in drinks easier). Rape involving non-violent factors can be just as traumatic for the victim as actual violence. The impact of date rape can have a profound effect on the victim's subsequent sex life, especially if he or she had lost the ability to offer resistance (drugged or physically subdued).

A problem for the male is that, from a social perspective, young men and women can see sexual coercion in dating or romantic situations as 'acceptable behaviour' and therefore the criminal consequences are not always self-evident.

Key points

- Despite an increasing awareness of the problem of sexual violence, there remains reluctance among some young men to recognise date rape as a criminal act or even unacceptable behaviour (Russo 2000).
- Date rape is rarely reported to the police and is generally under-reported.
- Date rape is an ambiguous crime because gender roles at the time of sexual contact make sexual consent a complex issue.
- Sexual consent is not always communicated clearly and is rarely witnessed.
- It is difficult to determine if verbal and emotional coercion (outside threats of violence) constituted an inappropriate coercion.
- Sexual consent is sometimes wrongly assumed for a wide range of reasons.

DOMESTIC VIOLENCE

Domestic violence has many forms, ranging from verbal abuse to repeated physical injury, it is neither haphazard nor a deviant behaviour. It is difficult to estimate the size of the problem because of the lack of suitable data. Nevertheless, broad estimates (using categories of violence listed below) suggest that domestic violence is widespread, almost to the point of being accepted as normal behaviour among some groups (Johnson & Ferraro 2000); and although not positively sanctioned in our society, it is at the very least tolerated in subtle ways.

Police are reluctant to be involved in what they continue to see primarily as a private family matter and while cognisant of their need to protect victims, at the same time must uphold the civil rights of the accused offender (Ellison 2002). Nurses are also placed in a similar position with the added difficulty of providing a standard of care to perpetrators and victims without prejudice. For most victims, the disclosure of abuse to the police or leaving a violent partner is a last resort. However, the victims are likely to confide in nurses soon after treatment and well informed nurses may play a key role in gathering information for referral to a domestic violence specialist. Routine enquiry by nurses for domestic violence can increase the rate of detection (Bacchus et al 2004).

Ironically, male perpetrators generally admit that violence per se is wrong. However, they deny responsibility for their personal actions by stating the violence was a justifiable action in response to a predisposing factor (wife did something wrong, alcohol consumption, their father was like this) or that they were out of control.

Knowledge of how to assist the perpetrators of violence is extremely limited and consequently there are few resources for men to turn to should they have insight into their problem or want to seek help. Separation has a devastating effect on violent men, as they are dependent on their spousal/de facto relationship. Consequently, this issue constitutes a major men's health problem and a challenge for the nurse.

Domestic violence can take many forms:

- Psychological and emotional abuse (personal degradation, feelings of incompetence)
- Verbal abuse (threats and harassment)
- Social abuse (forbidding spouse certain social contacts)
- Economic abuse (withholding financial resources)
- Sexual abuse (non consensual sexual intercourse).

Key points

- Men are the main perpetrators of violence.
- Many men who experienced violence as a child are no more likely than others to become perpetrators (the inverse is often assumed).
- Domestic violence transcends class and is embedded in many cultures.
- Non-physical forms of abuse can be as emotionally damaging as physical acts.
- Although offenders express remorse, a cycle of violence often ensues.
- Few men choose to seek help.

Women as perpetrators

In a review of historical data produced by the United States National Study of family violence conducted in 1975 and repeated in 1985, Mugford (1989) found that 'women are about as violent as men in the family'. This point was expanded upon in the sense that:

- Violence by men against women generally involves greater aggression, strength and impact
- Wife to husband violence often occurs in retaliation or self-defence
- Murdering of men by their spouse/partner usually occurs as a final response to years of domestic violence.

Cycle of violence

A cycle of violence model is useful in understanding what stage men who perpetrated violence are at when presenting for assessment:

- The build up to violence is self-generated within the man.
- The build up occurs regardless of spouse/partner responses.
- A violent outburst occurs followed by perpetrator remorse.
- Attempts are made to justify behaviours and assuage his guilt.
- The partner is pursued and subjected to displays of helplessness, often threats of suicide.
- If the man's emotional ploys are successful the violence abates and a honeymoon period or normalisation of the relationship ensues.

The cycle is likely to be repeated and become short-circuited. The short-circuiting occurs because the man somehow becomes increasingly insecure and dependent on the cycle.

Theoretical analysis

The causes of violence are complex and ideally the clinician aims for an integrated model. Approaches to understanding domestic violence include:

- Psychological theories on individual development and coping
- Social theories resulting from structural factors (family relations, demography)
- Sociocultural theories (emphasis on tradition and cultural traits)
- Feminist theories (hegemony and patriarchal societies).

Causes of violence

People in the general community are likely to view the causes of domestic violence in the following way:

- Unemployment
- Financial problems
- Gambling
- Heavy use of alcohol (related to stresses listed above)
- Unrealistic expectations of marriage
- Relationship pressures (sexist attitude at odds with spouse/partners needs)
- Jealousy
- Low self-esteem and inability to express self
- Inability to control anger.

Nursing issues

Spend some time considering your involvement in a domestic violence case:

- What are likely to be the attitudes of staff towards victims and perpetrators (will these attitudes contribute to better outcomes or simply reinforce stereotyping)?
- Explore your attitudes towards supporting a man who is the perpetrator of domestic violence.
- Consider your knowledge and the importance of confidential information.
- How do nurses develop a repertoire of questions to be asked at interview of a man accused of domestic violence (using non judgemental discourse)?
- What is your awareness of institutional procedures and protocols.
- What is your knowledge of national and local resources for victims.
- What is your knowledge of national and local resources for perpetrators.
- Identify ways to support men who are the victims of domestic violence.
- Identify legislation that affords protection for the victims of actual or potential violence.

Nursing issues—cont'd

- Be aware of violence issues associated with particular cultural norms among ethnic minorities.
- Health service intervention will not solve the problem; the aim is to provide supportive informed care and to direct perpetrators to appropriate referrals and resources.

CIRCUMCISION

Although medical circumcision of male infants for non-therapeutic reasons is legal in the UK and most countries, the Norwegian Council for Medical Ethics sees the procedure as a violent act and an affront to the child's human rights. Religious groups fervently defend the practice of routine circumcision.

The British Medical Association (BMA) has no policy on circumcision but guidelines (Committee on Medical Ethics 2003) are hotly debated in the British Medical Journal (Rickwood et al 2000, Singh 2003).

The British Association of Paediatric Surgeons (BAPS 1997, 2001) advises that there is rarely a clinical identification for circumcision. The American Medical Association (AMA 1999) supports the general principles of the 1999 Circumcision Policy Statement of the American Academy of Pediatrics (1995), making it clear that although there are potential benefits from circumcision, existing evidence is not sufficient to recommend routine neonatal circumcision.

Consent

The procedure is not essential to the newborn child's wellbeing, therefore a consent must be made on the basis of scientific evidence of the potential medical benefits weighed against the risks in the postoperative period. The BMA advises that consent must be given by parents in most cases of non-therapeutic circumcision.

Risks to male child

- Infection
- Haemorrhage
- Surgical mishap

- Adhesions
- Meatal stenosis
- Circumcision may be linked to erectile dysfunction.

The difficulty in gaining an informed consent lies in what weighting is applied to risk over the perceived medical and perceived social benefits.

Parents should be guided in their decision making on the basis of:

- Accurate information
- Unbiased presentation of information
- Opportunities to discuss issues.

Parental decisions may well be influenced by non-therapeutic, 'ritual' factors:

- Religious beliefs
- Circumcision is a physically defining feature in some religions
- Cultural/ethnic norms and practices
- Father's body image.

Nurses and doctors should take a non-judgemental approach to the decision of consent/non-consent to the procedure.

PREMATURE EJACULATION

When is ejaculation premature?

The term premature ejaculation lacks precision. Whether or not ejaculation is premature has to do with the man and his partner's preference for climax and is therefore a subjective concept. Lack of control over the timing of ejaculation/climax is the issue rather than 'premature ejaculation', or 'rapid ejaculation' as some sex counsellors are beginning to refer to the problem. Most men ejaculate 2–3 minutes after insertion of the penis (intromission).

Ejaculation is considered premature when it occurs:

- During initial foreplay
- At the time of insertion of the penis (vaginal intromission)
- Shortly after the insertion of the penis (intra-vaginal ejaculation).

A hypersensitive ejaculatory reflex affects approximately 40% of men and 30% of men aged between 40 and 70 years (Epperly & Moore 2000). Control over ejaculation timing appears to be a learned behaviour and one that can be learned incorrectly (reducing time to ejaculation). Incorrect behaviours can be reversed in most cases.

Causes

- Psychological factors that are postulated but not proven (relationship issues, performance anxiety), fear (unwanted pregnancy, being discovered 'in the act'), guilt (believing sexual intercourse is wrong/concerns over premarital sex/religious taboo)
- Physical problems (rare, e.g. prostate infection, urethritis)
- Neurological disorders (a rare cause)
- Sexual inexperience in learning to moderate arousal (a most likely cause)
- Problems within the relationship (a most likely cause).

Diagnosis

Diagnosis is by:

- Physical examination (usually no abnormalities detected)
- Interview with the man and his partner focusing on their relationship.

Helpful corrective techniques

- **Start and stop method** involves stopping of penis stimulation at a point where the man has not ejaculated, waiting approximately 30 seconds before resuming stimulation and continuing this process until ejaculation is desired.
- **The squeeze method** has had considerable success. The penis is stimulated and prior to ejaculation is squeezed where the shaft meets the glans at the head of the penis. After thirty seconds stimulation can be recommenced. The process is repeated until ejaculation is required.
- **Condoms** may also reduce the sensitivity of the penis and prolong the period from arousal to ejaculation.

Not so helpful techniques

- Distraction; some men try remembering sporting details during intercourse but this technique is of questionable value and results in less pleasure for the man.

- Although homeopathic creams, sprays and drops may be effective in the short term and may enhance self-esteem, they do not cure the problem.
- Couples should not simply read the literature and/or listen to lay advice and 'go it alone'. They should be directed to an accredited sexual health counsellor.

Treatments

Waldinger et al (2004) conducted a systematic review and meta-analysis of the efficacy of drug treatment of premature ejaculation. A meta-analysis of 35 daily treatment studies with selective serotonin reuptake inhibitors (SSRIs) and clomipramine demonstrated comparable efficacy of clomipramine with the SSRIs sertraline and fluoxetine in delaying ejaculation, However, the efficacy of the SSRI paroxetine was greater than all other SSRIs and clomipramine.

Various treatments can be tried:

- **Antidepressants** of the selective serotonin reuptake inhibitors (SSRIs) have, as a common side effect, the ability to prolong time to ejaculation. Those used for premature ejaculation are clomipramine, sertraline and fluoxethine. Low doses are normally given.
- **Local anaesthetic** creams are applied to the penis head to decrease sensation. Many men find that the pleasure of sex is reduced because of diminished sensation and there is the risk of transferring the effect to their partner's sensory receptors.
- **Counselling** with techniques proven to control the timing of sexual climax.

Is a cure possible?

With counselling, education and practice in techniques 95% of men with premature ejaculation are able to control their ejaculation. Couples first have to identify and resolve relationship issues so that they feel comfortable with each other. The central premise here is that without emotional intimacy, sexual relations are superficial and sexual problems such as premature ejaculation are rarely overcome. In addition, both partners need to consent to sexual intimacy without experiencing psychological pressure. Premature ejaculation is less likely if sexual activity occurs in a relaxed atmosphere and private space.

SEXUAL ABUSE

Child sexual abuse

Child sexual abuse is defined as unwanted sexual activity before the age of 18 years. Only a minority of children report abuse to their parents and only a minority of parents report abuse to the authorities. Whilst some families would prefer not to disclose abuse in order to protect the child, this is not an effective deterrent to perpetrators and children appreciate adults acting to protect them and other children.

Key points

- Men who were abused as children are more likely to become perpetrators of abuse.
- Child sexual abuse is more frequent in families beset by other adversity.
- Researchers predominantly focus on the victims' experiences, emotional anxieties and pathway to recovery.
- Few studies investigate why men sexually abuse children or the effects of rehabilitation programmes.
- There are a growing number of studies that recognise that women sexually abuse children.
- Variations in definitions of abuse, research methodologies and sampling differences have made it difficult to estimate the general prevalence of sexual abuse (ranges from 3% to 31%).
- People who report penetrative abuse in childhood have double the normal rates of mental disorders and suicide attempts (Andrews et al 2002).

Classification of severity

- Non-contact (sexual solicitation or exposure by an adult)
- Contact abuse (genital touching or fondling)
- Penetration (oral, anal, vaginal intercourse).

Perpetrators of assault are usually 'ordinary men' (relatives, family friends, trusted adults) and occasionally women. Although violence may be part of the assault, in many cases other techniques are employed to make a child take part in sexual activity (psychological threats, verbal threats, bribes, trickery).

Incidence

Sexual assault is more prevalent among young people under 25 years with 79% of sexual assault victims in Australia being female. In 61% of cases the assault was committed by a person known to the victim. One in four sexual assaults were perpetrated by a family member. Females were more likely than males who were abused to be assaulted by a stranger (Healey 2003). Australian police recorded 15 630 sexual assaults for the year 2000, representing 82 per 100 000 of the population. This represented an 11% increase since 1999 (Healey 2003).

Researching abused males

Holmes's (1998) synthesis of data from 166 American studies revealed a prevalence of male abuse ranging from 4% to 76%, depending on the definition of abuse. Holmes (1998) concluded that sexual abuse of boys appeared to be common, under-reported, under-recognised and under-treated. Several points emerged from this review of the research:

- Boys at risk were
  —< 13 years of age
  —Non-white
  —Living within lower socioeconomic groups
  —Not living with their father.
- Perpetrators were known but not related males.
- Abuse frequently occurred outside the home.
- Abuse involved penetration.
- Abuse occurred more than once.

Potential signs of sexual abuse

- Withdrawal from social contact/conversations
- Reluctance to go to school
- Sexual behaviour inappropriate for age
- Sexual play or drawing
- Complaints of pain, itching or injury to genital area
- Decline in school performance.

Emotional and psychological problems

1. Low self-esteem.
2. Sadness/depression.

3. Thought intrusion/nightmares.
4. Somatisation (headaches, dermatological problems).
5. Self-destructive behaviour.
6. Eating disorders.
7. Children may leave home prematurely to escape abuse.
8. Overuse of alcohol and other drugs is common in later life.

A review of studies of treatment for sexually abused children provides evidence to show that the sequelae listed above can be minimised, at least in the short term (Nurcombe et al 2000).

Nursing issues

Spend some time considering what you might tell children about sexual abuse in order to reduce the risk of the problem occurring. You may choose to explain that:

- Their body is their own and no one has the right to touch it in ways that make them scared.
- Grown ups sometimes do things that are not OK.
- A family member or friend might do something not OK.
- If someone touches them in a sexual way it is not their fault and they should tell someone.
- When adults talk openly about this problem and tell children what to do, it gives them permission to tell.

Implications for practice

- If you suspect child abuse or sexual abuse you must follow protocols within your organisation.
- In most places teachers, doctors, police and nurses are mandated notifiers.
- Be aware of any mandatory notifying procedures legislated within your county, state, province or country.
- You should be aware that nurses, midwives and school nurses should have been given child protection training with regular updates as part of their post registration education programme (Department of Health 1999).

> **Implications for practice—cont'd**
>
> • A child's ability to cope with sexual abuse once recognised or disclosed is strengthened by the support of a non-abusive adult carer who believes the child and is able to provide protection (Department of Health 1999).

How nurses should respond to the suspicion of abuse

• Record the child's details.
• Establish indicators of harm (reasons why you think abuse is possible).
• Make notes of physical and behavioural signs.
• Record date and time of observations.
• Carry out safety assessment (is the child in immediate danger?).
• Gather family information.
• Note cultural characteristics.
• Compose a reason for reporting (why call now?).
• Consult colleagues (advice and support).
• Develop an action plan based on organisational procedures.
• Talk to the child.

Sexually abused adult males

The notion that men can be victims of sexual abuse is relatively new. However, emerging research indicates that a significant minority of men were abused as children or raped as adults. Rape of an adult male is most often recorded within prisons and psychiatric clinics. The estimated prevalence by sex is 5.1% for males and 27.5% for females and this is comparable with other countries (Andrews et al 2002).

About 3% of American men – a total of 2.78 million men – have experienced an attempted or completed rape in their lifetime (National Institute of Justice Centers for Disease Control and Prevention 1998).

In 2002, one in every eight rape victims was male (Rennison & Rand 2002).

Whilst male rape is not uncommon in the prison system, it is difficult to quantify and prevent. Until the late 1990s very little attention was paid to the study of rape and sexual assault in male adulthood (Rentoul 1997). British law has only recently recognised this crime and in so doing has highlighted the need for specialist services for men. British empirical or other studies on male rape are limited and consequently it is difficult to identify, through evidence-based practice, the best practice for limiting the psychological consequences in the immediate period following the assault and in the long term.

References

American Academy of Pediatrics Committee on Bioethics 1995 Informed consent parental permission, and assent in pediatric practice. Pediatrics 95 (part 1): 314–317

American Medical Association 1999 Report 10 of the Council on Scientific Affairs (1–99). Online. available: http://www.ama-assn.org/ama/pub/category/13585.html

Andrews G, Gould B, Corry J 2002 Child sexual abuse revisited. [Editorial] Medical Journal of Australia 176(10): 458–459

Bacchus L, Mezey G, Bewley S et al 2004 Prevalence of domestic violence when midwives routinely enquire in pregnancy. British Journal of Obstetrics & Gynaecology, 111(5): 441

British Association of Paediatric Surgeons (BAPS) 1997 Statement an behalf of the British Association of Paediatric Surgeons concerning male ritual circumcision. Online. Available: http://www.baps.org.uk/documents/Circ%20GMC.html

British Association of Paediatric Surgeons (BAPS) 2001 Religious circumcision of male children: standards of care. Online. Available: http://www.cirp.org/library/statements/baps2/

Committee of Medical Ethics 2003 The law and ethics of male circumcision – guidance for doctors. British Medical Association, London

Department of Health 1999. The Protection of Children Act 1999: a practical guide to the Act for all organisations working with children. NHS Executive Department of Health London. Online. Available: http://www.dfes.gov.uk/publications/pdf/child protect.pd

Ellison L 2002 Prosecuting domestic violence without victim participation. Modern Law Review 65(6): 834

Epperly TD, Moore KE 2000 Health issues in men: part 1: common genitourinary disorders. American Family Physician 61(12): 3657–3664, 3547–3550

Healey J (ed) 2003 Sexual abuse. Issues in society Vol 179. Spinney Press

Holmes WC 1998 Sexual abuse of boys. The Journal of the American Medical Association 280(21):1855–1862

Johnson MP, Ferraro K 2000 Research on domestic violence in the 1990s: making distinctions. Journal of Marriage and Family 62(4): 948

Mugford J, 1989 Violence today. No. 2 Domestic Violence. Australian Institute of Criminology. Online. Available: http://www.aic.gov.au/publications/vt/vt2.html

National Institute of Justice Centers for Disease Control and Prevention (US Department of Justice) 1998 Prevalence, incidence and consequences of violence against women. National Institute of Justice, Washington, II DC

Nurcombe B, Wodding S, Marrington P et al 2000 Child sexual abuse 11: treatment. Australian and New Zealand Journal of Psychiatry 34(1): 92–97

Rennison CM, Rand R 2002 Criminal victimisation. National Crime Victimisation Survey. Bureau of Justice Statistics

Rentoul L 1997 Understanding the psychological impact of rape and serious sexual assault of men: a literature review. Journal of Psychiatric and Mental Health Nursing 4(4): 267

Rickwood AMK, Kenny SE, Donnell SC 2000 Towards evidence based circumcision of English boys: survey of trends in practice. British Medical Journal 321(7264): 792–793

Russo L 2000 Date rape: a hidden crime. Australian Institute of Criminology: Trends and issues in crime and criminal justice No. 157 (June). Online. Available: http://www.aic.gov.au/publications/tandi/ti157.pdf

Singh D 2003 BMA says non-therapeutic circumcision needs consent of both parents. British Medical Journal 326(7393): 782

Waldinger MD, Zwinderman AH, Schweitzer DH et al 2004 Relevance of methodological design for the interpretation of efficacy of drug treatment of premature ejaculation: a systematic review and meta-analysis. International Journal of Impotence Research 16(4): 369–381

Further reading

Anderson KL, Umberson D 2001 Gendering violence: masculinity and power in men's accounts of domestic violence. Gender and Society 15(3): 358–380.

Camino L 2000 Treating sexually abused boys: a practical guide for therapists and counsellors. Jossey-Bass, San Fransisco.

Dobash RE, Dobash RP 1998. Violent men and violent contexts. In: Dobash RE, Dobash RP (eds) Rethinking violence against women. Sage, Thousand Oaks, CA; p 141–168

Finkelhor D 1998 Improving research, policy and practice to understand child sexual abuse. Journal of the American Medical Association 280(21): 1864–1865

Gollaher DL 2000 Circumcision: a history of the world's most controversial surgery. Basic Books, New York

Hearn J 1998. The violence of men: how men talk about and how agencies respond to men's violence against women. Sage, Thousand Oaks, CA

Hobbs C 2002 Child protection in the United Kingdom: pediatric perspectives. Pediatrics International 44(5): 576–579

Peckover S 2002 Focusing upon children and men in situations of domestic violence: an analysis of the gendered nature of British health visiting. Health and Social Care in the Community 10(4): 254

Peckover S 2003 Health visitors' understandings of domestic violence. Journal of Advanced Nursing 44(2):200

Scully D 1990 Understanding sexual violence: a study of convicted rapists. Harper Collins Academic, London.

Chapter **8**

Male conditions and disorders

The conditions and disorders chosen for this handbook are those which are common and those which may be uncommon but can cause considerable distress to men. Men with uncommon conditions are likely to have little information on the topic.

HAEMATOSPERMIA (COMMON IN 'YOUNG MEN' LIFE PHASE)

Haematospermia is blood in ejaculate. This sign is likely to evoke fear and anxiety in young men and raise concerns about the possibility of malignancy. However, malignancy is a very rare cause but should be considered in men > 40 years. Long term follow-up shows no other serious problems arise (Shervington & Radcliffe 1993). This information should be used as a basis for reassuring men. A physical examination should be conducted on all men. Those men with other symptoms should have a full urological evaluation. However, in about 50% of cases the cause of haematospermia is not well understood.

Primary haematospermia

The term primary refers to the fact that there are no other symptoms. Although haematospermia can occur any time after puberty, the incidence peaks between 30 and 40 years.

- Approximately 15% of men have one episode.
- 85–90% of those who have haematospermia will have repeated episodes.
- Episodes are likely to become self-limiting.
- Usually begin treatment indicated if urinary symptoms are distressing.
- There is no risk of disease arising from haematospermia.
- There is no risk to the sexual partner.

Investigation

- Detailed history
- Physical examination (genital and rectal)
- Opportunity to screen for STIs
- Urinary examination (Narouz & Wallace 2002).

Secondary haematospermia

The term secondary refers to known causes of haematospermia (post prostate biopsy, urinary or prostate infection, cancer). Malignant cancers of the testicle and prostate are very rarely associated with haematospermia. Persistent haematospermia requires a referral to a urologist.

Urological evaluation when other symptoms are present

- Cystoscopy
- X-ray
- Ultrasound
- Rectal examination
- PSA and possible prostate biopsy.

DISORDERS OF THE PROSTATE

The prostate gland

The **location** of the gland is a fibromuscular organ positioned at the base of the bladder. It is a heart shaped structure 2.5 cm in length. This size is sustained until the age of 45 years when a second stage of growth begins. By the age of 65 some degree of urinary obstruction, related to prostate enlargement, is evident in most men. From the age of 70 years almost 90% of men show some sign of prostatic enlargement caused by hyperplasia (Nowak & Handford 1999).

The **function** of the prostate is not well understood. It secretes a thin, milky, alkaline fluid, which adds bulk to semen on ejaculation. It is thought that the alkaline characteristics may neutralise the acid environment of the vagina, thus promoting sperm motility and increasing the chances of fertilisation of an ovum. Sperm are not optimally mobile until surrounding fluids reach a pH of 6.0–6.5 and vaginal secretions a pH of 3.5–4.0.

Figure 8.1 identifies the prostate at the base of the bladder and surrounding the urethra. Enlargement of the prostate often results in a compression of the urethra and obstruction to the outward flow of urine. Urinary obstruction has the potential to cause a back flow of urine from the bladder, through the ureter(s), towards the kidneys. This backward flow can cause renal infection.

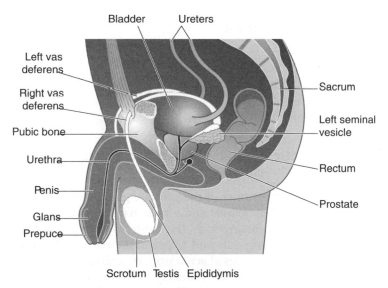

Figure 8.1   Male genito-urinary tract indicating site for prostate enlargement.

Prostatitis (common in maturity life phase)

Acute prostatitis is caused by a bacterial infection and can result in a febrile condition. On examination the gland is swollen, firm and very tender. Consequently, the examiner needs to be aware of the patient's level of comfort and digital palpation needs to be gentle. Chronic prostatitis does not produce consistent physical findings and therefore requires other methods of evaluation.

Treatment (acute phase)

Treatment usually consists of a course of antibiotics. Most antibiotics are unable to penetrate the gland because the low pH reduces the solubility of drugs. Non-bacterial induced prostatitis is difficult to treat and tends to be chronic. Treatment in the acute phase includes:

- Antibiotics
  —tetracycline
  —sulfamethoxazole combined with trimethoprim
- Stool softeners
- Rest
- Additional oral fluids.

Treatment (chronic phase)

- Prostatic massage
- Sexual activity resulting in ejaculation
- Anti-inflammatory agents
- Stool softeners
- Warm–hot sitz baths.

Benign prostatic hyperplasia (common in 'maturity' life phase)

The most common disorder of the prostate gland is benign prostatic hyperplasia (BPH). Whilst some texts refer to benign prostatic hypotrophy this is incorrect as the term hypertrophy refers to enlargement of existing cells and hyperplasia refers to the production of new tissue. Episodes of acute urinary retention are estimated at 1–2% and by the age of 80 years one in four men require treatment for symptoms attributed to BPH (Wilt 2002).

Incidence

BPH is apparent in approximately 8% of men in their fourth decade of life, reaching 70% by the seventh decade (Glynn 1985).

Signs and symptoms

Urological symptoms caused by BPH result in symptoms that are similar to, but not necessarily indicative of prostate cancer. Importantly, any man with lower urinary tract symptoms should be investigated by their GP (Sladden & Dickinson 1993, 1994). The following symptoms occur in 70% of men with BPH aged 70 years or more:

- Urgency to void
- Nocturia
- Weak stream
- Hesitancy with let down reflex
- Intermittency
- Incomplete emptying of the bladder.

Findings on examination by digital rectal examination (DRE)

- Firm though slightly elastic texture
- The gland usually feels smooth
- The median sulcus may be obliterated
- Most often there is unilateral enlargement (the gland may be symmetrically enlarged)
- Increased size.

N.B. BPH may obstruct the urethra even when general enlargement of the prostate has not been detected on examination.

Drug Treatment (Relaxes muscle in gland)

- alpha-blockers
- 5 alpha reductrase inhibitors (reduces gland size)

Prostate cancer (common in 'maturity' life phase)

Cancer of the prostate is the second most common malignancy among men (lung and colon tumours are first and second). However, more men die *with* prostate cancer than *from* it. This implies that, for the many men living with a diagnosis of prostate cancer, emotional and psychological support is essential to promote quality of life and avoid the co-morbidity of anxiety, neurosis and depression (Laws et al 2000).

Incidence

The UK has a crude incidence rate of 75 cases of prostate cancer per 100 000 with rates increasing steeply with increasing age. There are few cases registered in men aged under 50 years, and 95% of all cases occur in men over 60. One in 25 men (4%) will die from the disease. Trends in incidence rates may be misleading as cases of prostate cancer have increased as a result of a rise in PSA testing.

Men from Asia and the Far East have lower rates of prostate cancer relative to men in Europe; why this is so is not clear. The rates of prostate cancer rise in men who have migrated to countries where prostate cancer is more common (e.g. Japanese-Americans). This suggests that environmental factors contribute to risk factors (e.g. higher animal fat consumption).

Risk factors

- Strongest risk factor is age
- Ethnicity (Afro-Americans have high rate comparative to Caucasians)
- Family history of prostate cancer (first degree relative).

Clinical manifestations

Tumours of the prostate most often become manifest after the age of 50 years with a peak incidence emerging in the 70s. It is because many prostatic tumours arise near the periphery of the gland so that they cause little alteration to urinary flow and may remain undiscovered until pain is produced as a result of an invasion of cancerous tissue local to the gland.

Men with advanced disease may present with pain (especially back pain) resulting from widespread skeletal metastases. Any man experiencing urological symptoms should see his GP and may expect to be referred to a urologist.

General signs and symptoms

The symptoms for localised prostatic cancer may be the same as those for BPH but men often remain asymptomatic as many prostatic tumours arise near the periphery of the gland and as such do not immediately change urinary flow or voiding patterns. In this scenario prostatic tumours remain largely undiscovered until pain is produced as a result of an invasion of tissue local to the gland.

Most men with urological symptoms will be assessed using DRE and have a blood sample taken for PSA evaluation.

Findings on physical assessment (DRE)

- An area of hardness within the gland (may be a non cancerous formation)
- A distinct hard nodule that alters the gland's normal contour
- Irregularities that extend beyond the bounds of the gland
- The median sulcus may be obliterated.

(*For greater detail see section on DRE* in Chapter 9.)

Note that a raised PSA and findings outlined above (physical examination) do not in themselves support the diagnosis of cancer. Further investigations need to be conducted, usually a prostatic biopsy, and considered before the patient is informed of a definitive diagnosis. Even then, a biopsy may not detect an actual tumour because of the difficulty in accessing all parts of the gland.

Table 8.1 Stages of prostate cancer (Nowack & Handford 1999)

Stage	Substage	Clinical findings
A		No symptoms of tumour are found. A tumour is identified from biopsy
	A1	Microscopy identifies a low number of *well-differentiated* tumour cells
	A2	Microscopy identifies a large number of *poorly differentiated* cells
B		Tumour palpable via DRE. A mass is identified as being confined within the gland's capsule
	B1	A single mass is palpable
	B2	More extensive gland involvement
C		The invasion beyond capsule, based on evidence of local signs, symptoms and CT scan results
	C1	No invasion of the seminal vesicles
D		Evidence of metastases
	D1	Secondary spread is confined to pelvic lymph nodes
	D2	Metastases found in lung and/or bone

Stages of prostate cancer

A widely used system of stages of prostate cancer is based on a variety of clinical criteria and is shown in Table 8.1.

Treatments

Despite ongoing research and improving knowledge, new treatments that improve survival from prostate cancer remain elusive. Furthermore, there is no conclusive scientific evidence to show that any one treatment or combination of current treatments has a better survival outcome. No studies definitively support the benefits of aggressive treatment of clinically localised PC over watchful waiting after 10 years of follow up. Furthermore, 'radical prostatectomy and radiotherapy seem to be equally effective' (Austoker 1995). Using semi-structured interviews with men who had been treated for prostate cancer, Drummond et al (2001) determined that few could recall being informed of the differences in treatment options.

Patients are offered a range of treatments depending on age and the degree of advancement of the cancer.

Treatment choices

- Radiation therapy
- Radical prostatectomy
- Brachytherapy (radioactive pellets placed proximal to tumour site)
- Watchful waiting
- Hormone therapy
- Orchidectomy (castration).

Table 8.2 shows 10-year survival rates for three treatments.

In 1941 Charles Huggins demonstrated that castration changed the course of prostate cancer (Huggins 1972) and was awarded the Nobel prize for this breakthrough. However, few men choose surgical castration over chemical means. An orchidectomy is

Table 8.2 Treatment survival rates (Cancer stats 2002)

Treatment	10-year survival rate
Radical prostatectomy	80–90%
Radical radiotherapy	65–90%
Watchful waiting	70–90%

unpopular because of its quality of life effects. These include tiredness, impotence, loss of libido and hot flushes.

Men diagnosed with prostate cancer either have chemical treatments to reduce androgens or have an orchidectomy. This is because male hormones drive prostate cancers. Metastatic prostate cancer is first treated by androgen blockade but within a few months becomes hormone refractory.

Different treatments are discussed below:

- **Anti-androgens** (androgen receptor antagonists) suppress testicular and adrenal androgen production. An orchidectomy removes only 90% of circulating androgens; 10% emanate from the adrenals, making some chemical suppression necessary. There are two classes of androgen receptor antagonists, the non-steroidal (fultamide type) and steroidal (e.g. cyproterone acetate). Side effects from the non-steroidal type include gynaecomastia, affecting 20% of men, diarrhoea is experienced by approximately 15% and 3–5% develop liver function abnormalities. Potency and libido can be preserved in approximately 50% of men if monotherapy is employed effectively. The steroidal treatment carries an 8–10% risk of cardiovascular and cerebrovascular morbidity and can cause loss of libido, impotence and depression (Henry & O'Mahony 1999).
- **Oestrogen treatment** is effective in suppressing tumour growth; it is relatively inexpensive and has few side effects. However, this therapy carries the risk of gynaecomastia and breast pain (even at low doses) with two thirds of men experiencing these symptoms. Although effective in slowing the progress of the cancer, hormone manipulation is only a palliative treatment.
- **Luteinising hormone-releasing hormone** (LH-RH) is useful in the treatment of metastatic cancer and advanced cancer. However, it can cause a tumour surge because it initially triggers testosterone production. It is therefore recommended that cyproterone acetate be given 3–7 days prior to LH-RH. This treatment requires parenteral administration. LH-RH is expensive compared with an orchidectomy, has similar survival outcomes and the duration of response is limited to 18 months.
- **Radiation therapy** offers equivalent survival rates to radical surgery. Radiotherapy is given as a palliative measure by hemibody irradiation or spot radiation for treatment of metastatic foci within bones. The treatment is usually complete in 6–7 weeks. Disease-free survival for stage A is 83% (5 years) and

67% (10 years) and for stage B survival is 70% and 51% respectively over the same time frame.

- **Brachytherapy** involves the implantation of radioactive seeds into the prostate gland. The implantation occurs transrectally, guided by ultrasound or CT scan, and is a day surgery procedure. The seeds remain in situ permanently, providing an intense dose of radiation to specific tissue. This is a relatively inexpensive means of offering effective radiotherapy. There are few side effects; provided the peri-ureteral tissue is avoided, the complication of urethritis is unlikely and impotence is uncommon (Henry & O'Mahony 1999).

Watchful waiting

Little is know about the natural progression of prostate cancer beyond 10–15 years of watchful waiting. A longitudinal study conducted in Sweden (Johansson et al 2004), spanning some 20 years and involving 223 men, is the largest and longest of its type. The study has revealed that mortality increased from 15:1000 to 44:1000 and that the disease accelerates after 15 years, regardless of the stage at which the tumour was first diagnosed. The main conclusion is that:

> Although most prostate cancers diagnosed at an early stage have an indolent course, local tumor progression and aggressive metastatic disease may develop in the long term. These findings would support early radical treatment, notably among patients with an estimated life expectancy exceeding 15 years. (Johansson et al 2004, p. 2713)

Radical prostatectomy

The commonest treatment for prostate cancer and benign prostatic hyperplasia is transurethral resection of the prostate (TURP). This procedure is covered in detail in Chapter 9.

TESTICULAR CANCER ('PRIME TIME' LIFE PHASE)

Epidemiology

Testicular carcinoma is the most common malignancy among men aged between 15 and 34 years (Abbas et al 2002), accounting for 20% of all cancer in Caucasian males between the ages of 20 and 35 years (Algood et al 1988). Scottenfield et al (1980) reported that during the 40-year period 1936–1976 the incidence of testicular cancer (TC) doubled. Silverberg (1985) also noted that between 1975 and 1985 the probability of a male child developing TC had doubled. The overall incidence of TC has been steadily rising with an increase of 15–20% being observed in successive 5-year periods (Cancer Research Campaign 1998).

Populations at risk

In the US testicular cancer occurs infrequently among African-Americans and the native Japanese population. Caucasian males have a four-fold greater risk of a diagnosis of testicular cancer compared to their African-American males (Lantz et al 2001). The highest incidence occurs among Caucasian men in northern Europe (Dearnaley et al 2001, p. 1583). A social gradient has also been observed with working class males having a relatively lower incidence of testicular cancer than professionals and those in higher social class (Algood et al 1988).

At risk groups

Testicular cancer has a low but definite familial occurrence (Algood et al 1988). However, the overall incidence of a positive family history in TC is very low, only 2%. Dearnalcy et al (2001) report that siblings of men with TC are 6–10 times more likely to develop the cancer. The most important risk factor is testicular maldescent of testes (Dearnaley et al 2001). Whilst a strong correlation exists between TC, testicular maldescent and testicular abnormalities, it remains uncertain whether these are a cause in themselves or share similar environmental or genetic factors.

Risk factors for TC

- History of cryptorchidism (well established risk)
- Undescended testes
- Testicular trauma (within 2 years of diagnosis)
- Having had a sexually transmitted disease.

There is no support for increased risk related to:

- elevated testicular temperature (tight jeans or underwear)
- occupational factors
- TC after vasectomy (Moller et al 1994).

Clinical manifestations

Testicular tumours, in most cases, present as:
- A painless intrascrotal lump, swelling or enlargement
- A hard lump on the front or side of the testicle
- A dragging inguinal pain caused by the increased weight of the enlarged testis (swelling)
- A dull ache in lower stomach, groin or scrotum
- Increase in firmness in one testicle
- Asymmetry within the testis
- Back pain (less common and associated with para-aortic lymph node metastases.

Abnormal masses in the epididymis are common but likely to be associated with a testicular tumour. Tumours that grow rapidly may cause a substantial degree of pain and discomfort.

Nursing assessment in suspected TC

More than 90% of men with TC present with scrotal symptoms. In cases of a rapidly growing tumour a two-handed examination of the intrascrotal contents is recommended as it will assist in differentiating a mass within the testis from one within the epididymis (Hayden 1993). The tumour itself usually presents as firm and symmetrical. Typically, the application of pressure to the enlarged testis does not tend to produce pain. A more accurate assessment of the nature of an intrascrotal mass is gained with ultrasound and the tumour markers serum alpha-fetoprotein, human chorionic gondatrophin (HCG) and lactic dehydrogenase (LHDH) (Hayden 1993, p. 1358).

Aetiology

The cause of TC is unknown. Although numerous factors have been proposed for the aetiology of testicular cancer, only a history of cryptorchidism correlates strongly. All the risk factors suggested in the literature were explored in a study carried out across nine health regions in England (Anonymous 1994).

Factors contributing to testicular cancer

- Gynaecomastia may be present in pre-adolescent boys; there may also be virilisation (Holleb et al 1991 found in Lantz et al 2001).

- Testicular trauma, at least 2 years prior to diagnosis, was associated with an odds ratio (OR) of 2.00 (if the odds ratio is approximately one, then this is evidence of no difference in risk for having this injury).
- Having ever had a sexually transmitted disease was also associated with an increased risk) (OR = 2.22).
- There were no clear occupational associations and there was no association with scrotal temperature (hot baths, type of underpants, jeans). (Anonymous 1994)

Survival rates

Between 50 and 60% of TC cases are seminoma and 30% of cases are teratoma. Survival from metastatic teratoma has increased from 20% (1970s) to at least 90% (mid 1990s). However, those cases exhibiting large metastatic disease from teratoma have approximately a 60% survival rate (Austoker 1995).

Prior to the development of effective chemotherapy in the 1970s, less than 10% of men with metastatic non-seminomatous germ cell tumours were cured; nowadays approximately 90% are potentially cured (Peckham 1988).

Diagnosis

It is not possible to take a biopsy of testicular tissue because of the uncertainty that tumour tissue can be located in the tissue sample. Consequently, surgery is undertaken with the prospect of removing the testicle and a biopsy is performed in the first stage of surgery. A tissue sample is sent immediately to a pathologist and if cancer is confirmed then the testicle is removed. Normally it will be reasonably certain that the testicle contains a tumour.

Treatment options

If the cancer is detected in the early stages of its development and there are no signs of metastases surgery may be the only treatment. Some centres/physicians use radiotherapy post surgery for forms of cancer that are very responsive to this kind of treatment (seminomas). Some physicians/centres have a policy of watchful waiting. Men should be offered the option of storing their semen prior to surgery in the event that fertility is diminished or infertility occurs. It is possible to have a testicular prosthesis fitted (silicone based) to reduce the prospect of altered body image, however, this option is rarely taken up. Where a tumour has spread to the lymph nodes (usually those to the posterior of the abdomen), a lymphectomy is performed and chemotherapy may be recommended.

Survival

TC's responsiveness to chemotherapy containing platinum has meant that 95% of men with TC can expect a cure (Dearnaley et al 2001). Approximately 5% of men who have been cured (5 year survival without occurence) of TC develop a tumour in their remaining testicle. Although 6900 new cases of testicular cancer were projected to occur in 2000, only 300 men were expected to die as a result of the disease (American Cancer Society 2000).

Survival defined

Survival refers to the percentage of people still alive 1, 3, 5 and 10 years after they have been diagnosed with cancer. The 5-year survival rate is often quoted. *Relative survival* takes into account the fact that the person may have died even if he did not have cancer; it is relative to the rest of the population. 5-year relative survival for men for all cancers combined (excluding non-melanoma skin cancer (NMSC) and a few very rare cancers) is approximately 31% for England and Wales for patients diagnosed between 1986 and 1990. For women it is approximately 43%. (See Cancer Research UK website. Statistics. http://www.cancerresearchuk.org/aboutcancer/statistics/survival?version=1)

Nursing issues

Consider evidence based strategies for supporting men with a diagnosis of TC:

- What concerns might men raise regarding their survival?
- Have these men considered fathering children in the future?
- Are these men concerned about alterations in sexual function?
- Do the issues men hold in relation to their diagnosis and treatment have the potential to alter their:
  - emotional and psychological wellbeing to the extent that it interferes with their sex life
  - self-image (e.g. masculinity)?

Nursing issues—cont'd

N.B. It may be difficult to locate suitable information on men's concerns. If that is the case it is recommended that you access the Clinical Oncology Information Network (COIN) guidelines (COIN 2000) and Laws (1998).

References

Abbas K, Oakeshott P 2002 Pilot study of testicular cancer awareness and testicular self examination in men attending two south London general practices. Family Practice 19(3): 294–296

Algood CB, Newell GR, Johnson DE 1988 Viral etiology of testicular tumours. Journal of Urology 139(2): 308–310

American Cancer Society 2000 Testicular cancer. What is it? In: Cancer Resource Centre. Online. Available: http://www.cancer.org/docroot/CRI/CRI_2_3x.asp?dt=41

Anonymous 1994 [Page No. 8/14] British Journal of Cancer 70(3): 513–520

Austoker J 1995 Cancer prevention in primary care: screening for ovarian, prostatic, and testicular cancer. British Medical Journal 309(6950): 315–320

Cancer Research Campaign 1998 Testicular cancer: fact sheet 16. Cancer Research Campaign, London

Cancer stats (February 2002) Cancer Research UK

Clinical Oncology Information Network (COIN) 2000 Guidelines on the management of adult testicular cancer. Clinical Oncology 12(Suppl): S173–S210

Dearnaley DP, Huddart RA, Horwich A 2001 Managing testicular cancer. British Medical Journal 322(7302): 1583–1588

Drummond MJ, Laws TA, Poljak-Fligic J 2001 Knowledge and attitudes towards prostate cancer among Italo-Australian men. Australian Journal of Primary Health Interchange 7(3): 9–16

Glynn RJ, Campion EW, Bouchard GR et al 1985 The development of benign prostatic hyperplasia among volunteers in the Normative Aging Study. American Journal of Epidemiology 121(1): 78–90

Hayden LJ 1993 Chronic testicular pain. Australian Family Physician 22(8): 1357–1365

Henry RY, O'Mahony D 1999 Treatment of prostate cancer. Journal of Clinical Pharmacy and Therapeutics 24: 93–102

Holleb A, Fink D, Murphy G 1991 American Cancer Society textbook of clinical oncology. American Cancer Society, Atlanta

Huggins C 1972 Nobel lectures. Physiology of medicine 1963–1970. Elsevier, Amsterdam. Online. Available: http://www.nobelprize.org/medicine/laureates/1966/huggins-bio.html

Johansson JE, Andrén O, Andersson SO et al 2004 Natural history of early localized prostate cancer. JAMA 291(22): 2713–2719

Lantz JM, Fullerton JT, Harshburger RJ et al 2001 Promoting screening and early detection of cancer in men. Nursing and Health Science Journal 3(4): 189–196

Laws TA 1998 Testicular cancer: Michael's story. In: Laws TA (ed) Promoting men's health: an essential book for nurses. Ausmed Publications, Melbourne

Laws TA, Drummond M, Polijak-Flijak J 2000 On what basis do Australian men make informed decisions about diagnostic and treatment options for prostate cancer? Australian Journal of Primary Health Interchange 6(2): 86–93

Moller H, Knudesen LB, Lynge E 1994 Risk of testicular cancer after vasectomy: cohort study of over 73 000 men. British Medical Journal 309(6950): 295–299

Narouz N, Wallace DM 2002 Haematospermia in the context of a genitourinary medicine unit. International Journal of STD and AIDS 13(8): 517–521

Nowak TJ, Handford AG 1999 Essentials of pathophysiology. McGraw-Hill, Dubuque, IA

Peckham M 1988 Testicular cancer. Acta Oncologica 27(4): 439–453

Scottenfield M, Warshauer E, Sherlock S et al 1980 The epidemiology of testicular cancer in young adults. American Journal of Epidemiology 112(2): 232–246

Shervington J, Radcliffe KW 1993 Haematospermia [Comment]. International Journal of STD and AIDS 3(5): 313–315

Silverberg E 1985 Cancer statistics. CA: a cancer journal for clinicians 35(1): 19–45

Sladden M, Dickinson J 1993 Effectiveness of screening for prostate cancer. Australian Family Physician 22(8): 1385–1392

Sladden M, Dickinson J 1994 Carcinoma of the prostate. The Medical Journal of Australia 160: 310–311

Wilt TJ 2002 Treatment options for benign prostatic hyperplasia. British Medical Journal 324(7345): 1047–1048

Further reading

Amir V, Kaisary AV, Murphy GP et al 2000 Textbook of prostate cancer: pathology, diagnosis and treatment. Martin Dunitz, [Page no. 8/17]

Davies JM 1981 Testicular cancer in England and Wales: some epidemiological aspects. Lancet 1(8226): 928–932

Fernand L, Koutsillieris M 2004 Prostate cancer: understanding the pathophysiology and re-designing a therapeutic approach. McGraw-Hill Professional,

Gottlieb S 2000 Impotence more common after prostatectomy than previously thought. British Medical Journal 320(7230): 272

Henry RY, O'Mahany D 1999 Treatment of prostate cancer. Journal of Clinical Pharmacy and Therapeutics 24: 93–102

Institute of Cancer Research 2001 Men still dangerously ignorant about male cancers. The Institute of Cancer Research, London, UK. *Specialises in basic and clinical research, training and education.* http://www.icr.ac.uk/press/releases/mori.html

Jakobsson L, Hallberg IR, Loven L 1997 Experiences of daily life and life quality in men with prostate cancer. An explorative study. Part I. European Journal of Cancer Care 6(2): 108–116

Jakobsson L, Loven L, Hallberg IR 2001 Sexual problems in men with prostate cancer in comparison with men with benign prostatic hyperplasia and men from the general population. Journal of Clinical Nursing 10(4): 573–582

Khadra A, Oakeshott P 2002 Pilot study of testicular cancer awareness and testicular self-examination in men attending two South London general practices. Family Practice 19(3): 294–296

Laguna MP, Pizzocaro G, Klepp O et al 2001 EAU Working Group on Oncological Urology. EAU guidelines on testicular cancer. European Urology 40(2): 102–110

MORI poll 1999 Awareness of testicular and prostate cancer. Institute of Cancer Research http://www.mori.com/polls/1998/menshlth.shtml

Chapter **9**

Procedures and investigations

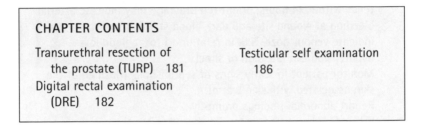

TRANSURETHRAL RESECTION OF THE PROSTATE (TURP)

Cancerous tissue and tissue from benign prostatic hyperplasia are commonly scraped away via a cystoscopy approach. A spinal anaesthetic is preferred, particularly for older men who are a poor surgical risk.

Indications for using surgical approaches other than transurethral are prostate weight > 40 g, where there is severe urethral stricture or where there are joint problems reducing the degree of flexion, thus posing difficulty in positioning of the patient for a cystoscope.

Alternative methods of removing prostate tissue are:

- Suprapubic transvisceral (abdominal incision using bladder entry)
- Retropubic extravesical (low abdominal incision without bladder entry).

Postoperative care for this procedure is described in Box 9.1.

It is important that nurses who do not experience at first hand the care of men with prostate problems and TURP, gain an

---

Box 9.1 Postoperative care for men having TURP

- Continuous bladder irrigation will be in operation.
- Traction may have been in place on the urinary catheter to prevent haemorrhage; review orders to determine when that may be released (may cause bladder spasm and discomfort).
- Bladder spasm can occur from pressure of the catheter's balloon on the bladder neck or clots reducing the free drainage of urine and irrigation fluid (check bladder size by judicious abdominal palpation; if the bladder is enlarged then inform physician of the possible need for bladder irrigation).
- Expect the urine to move to a blood–tinged colour and consistency within 24 hours; bright red drainage may indicate arterial bleeding at wound site and dark blood staining with clots may indicate venous ooze. N.B. In relation to total blood loss, hypotension is a late sign of shock.
- Monitor patient for early signs of septic shock (flushing of the skin associated with skin warmth).
- Report abnormal findings promptly.
- If bleeding becomes substantial then monitor the patient for disseminated intravascular coagulation (DIC) resulting from the release of large amounts of tissue thromboplastin.
- Do not insert instruments into the rectum (e.g. temperature probes, enema tubes).
- Ensure there are orders to prevent constipation to minimise the risks of straining during defecation and putting pressure on the prostatic capsule.

---

understanding of the complexity of factors that affect these men. The works listed in the "Further Reading" section at the end of this chapter are excellent examples of efforts to gain understanding of the factors and the richness of the data relating to these men's lived experiences vis a vis treatment for prostate cancer.

DIGITAL RECTAL EXAMINATION (DRE)

DREs are conducted for several reasons: they can aid in the detection of cancer of the rectum and are used to palpate the prostate. When the intention is to palpate the prostate the opportunity should not be missed to examine other structures for abnormalities.

Procedure

- A flexible light source is required.
- Wash and warm your hands.
- Glove your hand.
- Index finger should be lubricated.
- Men should stand, flex forward at the hips and rest their elbows and arms on an examination couch with knees slightly apart.
- Part the buttocks and ask the patient to bear down/strain, then inspect the anus (note any inflammation, skin tags, scars, fissures, haemorrhoids, swelling, excoriation or mucosal bulging).
- Have a paper towel at hand to remove lubricant or any faecal material once the finger is gently withdrawn at the close of the examination.

Technique (anal and rectal examination)

- Place the pad of the index finger against the anal sphincter.
- Ask the patient to bear down/strain.
- Once the sphincter relaxes slowly insert the finger and point it towards the patient's umbilicus.
- If the sphincter remains taut, reassure the patient that he will experience only minor discomfort and retry insertion.
- Do not force an insertion of the finger.
- He may feel as if he were moving his bowels, reassure him that this will not occur.
- Ask the patient if there is any discomfort (normally minimal).
- Note that the sphincter should contract evenly around the finger.
- Rotate the finger (clockwise then counter-clockwise) around the musculature of the anal ring to assess its characteristics.
- Then insert the finger as far as possible to palpate the rectal wall (discomfort should be minimal).

Document as abnormal findings if:

- surface abnormalities are apparent (haemorrhoids are the most common abnormality)
- the sphincter did not tighten evenly
- nodules or a mass are detected
- there is obvious localised or general tenderness
- irregularities in the anal ring or rectum are evident
- polyps are found.

Technique (palpating the prostate gland)

After sweeping the wall of the rectum (clockwise then anticlockwise) return to the midline and turn your body somewhat away from the patient more easily to feel the prostate. Palpate the anterior rectal surface to assess the posterior surface of the prostate. The patient may state that he feels the urge to urinate. Reassure him that this is a sensation only and that he will not pass water. Sweep your finger carefully over the prostate gland, identifying its lateral lobes and the medial sulcus between them. If possible, extend your finger above the gland to the region of the seminal vesicles and the peritoneal cavity.

Figure 9.1 shows how the prostate is palpated at the time of DRE. This procedure is also used to detect cancer of the rectum and lower bowel.

The characteristics of a *normal* prostate gland, as palpable through the anterior rectal wall, are:

- Smooth in consistency
- Non-tender
- Firm but not hard
- Slightly mobile
- Symmetrical and bilobal in contour
- Median sulcus can be felt between two lateral lobes
- Diameter one and a half inches (3.8 cm)
- Projecting less than half an inch (1 cm) into the rectum.

Note that only the posterior wall of the gland is palpable.

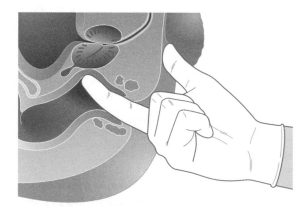

Figure 9.1   Digital rectal examination.

Documenting the size of the prostate

Some indication of the size of the prostate gland can be gained by estimating the extent of its protrusion into the rectum. Thompson and Wilson (1996) suggest grades can be allocated according to the depth of protrusion.
Protrusion of:

- < 1 cm is expected
- 1–2 cm is grade 1
- 2–3 cm is grade 2
- 3–4 cm is grade 3
- 4 cm or > is grade 4

Document as *abnormal* findings if:

- there is tenderness
- there is asymmetry in the contour
- the median sulcus is not obvious or obliterated
- if there is an irregular surface consisting of nodules
- a boggy consistency (may be indicative of benign prostatic hyperplasia)
- a rock hard prostate (may be indicative of carcinoma or calculi or fibrosis).

Findings in prostate cancer

- An area of hardness within the gland (may be a non-cancerous formation)
- A distinct hard nodule that alters the gland's normal contour
- Irregularities that extend beyond the bounds of the gland
- The median sulcus may be obliterated.

Note that a raised PSA and findings outlined above (physical examination) do not in themselves support the diagnosis of cancer. Further investigations, usually a prostatic biopsy, need to be conducted, and considered before the patient is informed of a definitive diagnosis. Even then, a biopsy may not detect an actual tumour because of the difficulty in accessing all parts of the gland.

Findings in benign prostatic hyperplasia (BPH)

- Firm though slightly elastic texture
- The gland usually feels smooth.

- The median sulcus may be obliterated.
- The gland may be symmetrically enlarged.

Size may not be a good indicator of the extent of hyperplasia. Although general enlargement may not be detectable on examination, there could be local encroachment on the urethral wall, causing diminished stream of urine or difficulty in commencing micturition.

Findings in acute prostatitis

Acute prostatitis is caused by a bacterial infection and can result in a febrile condition. On examination the gland is swollen, firm and very tender. Consequently, the examiner needs to be aware of the patient's level of comfort and digital palpation needs to be gentle. Chronic prostatitis does not produce consistent physical findings and therefore requires other methods of evaluation.

TESTICULAR SELF EXAMINATION

Many men will have heard about testicular self examination as a means of detecting testicular cancer. Aside from the debate on using this form of assessment as a screening method, nurses should be able to instruct men on the procedure because it could help confirm concerns men may have about abnormal sensations (pain, dragging feeling) in their testes. Testicular cancer is identifiable in early stages through self-examination and this is recommended at 4-weekly intervals (Lantz et al 2001).

The use of TSE in the following manner is likely to prompt men to seek medical advice should they detect an abnormality:

- Ideally the testes should be warm on examination (after shower or bath).
- Note that normally one testis is slightly bigger than the other and the left hangs lower.
- Support the scrotum with the palm of the non-dominant hand.
- Gently roll one of the testes between the thumb and forefinger of the dominant hand.
- The testis should feel firm and smooth.
- Feel for any lumps or swelling on the surface of the testicles.
- Using thumb and forefinger, feel under the skin at the rear of the testis for the epididymis. This highly coiled tube carrying

sperm to the vas deferens should be soft to the touch. Check for swelling of the epididymis.
- Repeat this procedure with the other testis.

Readers should refer to Figure 2.2a and 2.2b in Chapter 2.

References

Lantz JM, Fullerton JT, Harshburger RJ et al 2001 Promoting screening and early detection of cancer in men. Nursing and Health Science Journal 3(4): 189–196
Thomson J, Wilson S 1996 Health assessment for nursing practice. Mosby, Philadelphia

Further reading

Callaghan P, Yuk-Lung C, King-Yu Ida Y et al 1998 Evidence-based care of Chinese men having transurethral resection of the prostate (TURP). Journal of Advanced Nursing 28(3): 576
Gottlieb S 2000 Impotence more common than previously thought. British Medical Journal 320(7230): 272
Jakobsson L 2002 Indwelling catheter treatment and health-related quality of life in men with prostate cancer in comparison with men with benign prostatic hyperplasia. Scandinavian Journal of Caring Sciences 16(3): 264–271
Jakobsson L, Hallberg IR, Loven L 1997 Experiences of daily life and life quality in men with prostate cancer. An explorative study. Part I. European Journal of Cancer Care 6(2): 108–116
Jakobsson L, Hallberg IR, Loven L 2000 Experiences of micturition problems, indwelling catheter treatment and sexual life consequences in men with prostate cancer. Journal of Advanced Nursing 31(1): 59–67
Jakobsson L, Loven L, Hallberg IR 2001 Sexual problems in men with prostate cancer in comparison with men with benign prostatic hyperplasia and men from the general population. Journal of Clinical Nursing 10(4): 573–582
Jakobsson L, Loven L, Hallberg IR 2004 Micturition problems in relation to quality of life in men with prostate cancer or benign prostatic hyperplasia: comparison with men from the general population. Cancer Nursing 27(3): 218–229
Moore KN, Estey A 1999 The early post-operative concerns of men after radical prostatectomy Journal of Advanced Nursing 29(5): 1121–1129
Pateman B 2000 Men's lived experience following transurethral prostatectomy for benign prostatic hyperplasia. Journal of Advanced Nursing 31(1): 51
Templeton H, Coates VE 2001 Adaptation of an instrument to measure the informational needs of men with prostate cancer. Journal of Advanced Nursing 35(3): 357

Chapter **10**

Male-specific conditions and disorders

The conditions for review in this chapter have been selected on the basis that they cause significant morbidity if left undiagnosed or incorrectly diagnosed. Types of morbidity include strangulation of the bowel (hernia), infarction of the testis (testicular torsion) and reduction or absence of fertility (orchitis, epididymitis). These problems can be detected early by nurses who are informed on men's health problems, have a clear understanding of the male anatomy and can perform a systematic physical assessment. Any of the conditions discussed in this chapter, if diagnosed by the nurse, will require prompt referral to a medical doctor.

A diagram such as Figure 10.1 should be used to orientate the male patient to an understanding of the structures affected by any one of the common conditions outlined in this chapter.

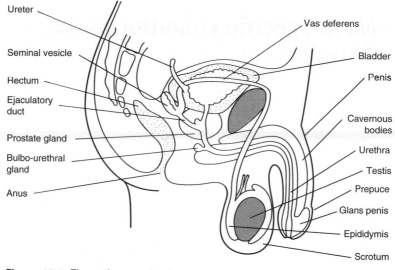

Figure 10.1 The male reproductive system.

HYDROCELE

Hydroceles are scrotal swellings caused by a collection of fluid in the scrotal sac. In infants approximately 90% of these will resolve spontaneously (Davenport 1996a). In children (1–2 years) most hydroceles are congenital. The incidence of hydrocele is 1% in adult males.

Hydroceles occurring in an adult usually have a secondary cause:

- Traumatic (haemorrhagic) causes are common
- Infection
- Effects of radiotherapy
- Testicular torsion (Pentyala et al 2001)
- After renal transplantation.

Implications for practice

The following points are requisite knowledge for nurses who are assisting in the diagnosis of an enlarged scrotum and supporting the patient in his understanding of the problem and treatment options.

On examination

Hydroceles are usually bilateral, and easily detected by the health professional. They are located superior and anterior to the testis whilst spermatoceles lie superior and posterior to the testis. Unless an infection causes an acute hydrocele, no erythema or scrotal discoloration is observed. The hydrocele is larger and relatively tense after prolonged standing. The size usually decreases when the patient is made recumbent. Gentle palpation of the testis should be performed because of the possibility of testicular tumour. 70% of renal transplant patients have a hydrocele on the same side as the new kidney. A focused light source will shine clearly through the fluid-filled sac. Transillumination occurs in hydrocele and incursion of the bowel (hernia). As hydroceles and hernias have a similar anatomy, a differential diagnosis is required (see section on inguinal hernia). It is estimated that in 20% of adult patients presenting with hydrocele, testicular torsion is the cause. The clinician or nurse may be misled by focusing on the hydrocele, which delays the diagnosis of torsion.

At interview

- Most men present with a painless, enlarged scrotum.
- Genito-urinary symptoms are absent in uncomplicated hydrocele.
- Some men experience a dragging sensation in the scrotal region.
- Occasionally, a mild discomfort radiating along the inguinal area to the mid portion of the back is reported (Pentyala et al 2001).

There may be a history of:

- Trauma
- Radiotherapy
- Local infection (orchitis or epididymitis)
- Systemic infection (tuberculosis and tropical disease).

Laboratory tests

- Complete blood picture (may indicate an inflammatory/infective process)
- Scrotal ultrasound may detect tumour, hernia (incarcerated bowel or spermatocele)
- Doppler may be used to detect blood flow in the case of testicular torsion or severe trauma.

Treatment

Aspiration of the hydrocele is not recommended because:

1. It introduces a portal of entry for microorganisms (infection).
2. As many as 50% of acute hydroceles of the scrotum are misdiagnosed (torsion of the testis, hernias). Perforation of the bowel will occur if a hernia is undetected.
3. Consult a urologist if hernia, testicular mass or testicular torsion is suspected.

Surgical repair

The nurse should ensure that an informed consent occurs. The patient should be made aware that surgery can result in:

- Injury to the vas deferens (fertility problems)
- Infection rates of 2%
- Direct injury to spermatic vessels
- Postoperative haemorrhagic hydrocele (not uncommon but should resolve quickly).

TESTICULAR TORSION

Adolescents have the highest prevalence of acute scrotal pathology. The most important disorders in this group are torsion of the testes and acute epididymitis. Torsion is the most common acute disorder of the testes in children and young adults. Testicular torsion is a twisting of the spermatic cord that supports the testes. The twisting encroaches on testicular blood supply and an infarction can ensue. The possibility of infarction makes accurate diagnosis and timely surgical intervention paramount. Patients have been treated for epididymitis (with antibiotics) when the correct diagnosis was torsion of the tests, thus making differential diagnosis very important (Davenport 1996b).

Differential diagnosis

- Doppler ultrasound examination (without delay)
- Urgent radionuclide scrotal imaging (cost effective and accurate)
- If there is doubt, a surgical exploration should be considered mandatory (Davenport 1996b, Luscombe 1996).

At interview

Patients will report:
- Sudden onset of acute pain
- Pain radiating into the groin
- Some nausea and possibly vomiting.

On examination

- Testicle is swollen
- Testis is draw upward or even horizontal
- The scrotum become red and oedematous.

Surgical treatment

As the anatomical abnormality predisposing to torsion is commonly bilateral, both testes should be surgically fixed in the normal anatomical position (non-dissolving sutures). All patients should be followed up as outpatients as there is an incidence of late-onset testicular atrophy. Successful aversion of testicular ischaemia/infarction relies on minimising the time between the onset of symptoms and surgery (Davenport 1996b). A testicular prosthesis (silicone) is an option for those who have had an infarcted testicle removed (orchidectomy).

EPIDIDYMITIS

Epididymitis is an acute inflammatory process that occurs most commonly in young adult males. The inflammation is the result of an ascending infection from the ejaculatory duct, through the vas deferens and into the epididymis. Epididymitis in adolescents and young adults is often related to sexual activity and *does not* present with a urinary tract infection. The source of the infection is usually *Chlamydia trachomatis* or *Neisseria gonorrhoea* (sexually transmitted). However, in pre-pubertal males, epididymitis is almost always associated with a urinary tract anomaly (Galejs & Kass 1999).

Implications for practice

Prompt and accurate diagnosis is essential because inflammation and collection of fluid in the scrotal sac can impede blood flow to reproductive organs.

On examination

- Noticeable swelling on one or both sides of scrotum
- Severe pain and tenderness in the scrotum
- The patient guards the scrotum when walking
- The patient may be unable to ambulate because of pain
- A urethral discharge may be present.

Tests

- Urinalysis shows elevated white blood cell (WBC) count.
- Culturing of urine shows presence of bacteria.
- Epididymitis accompanied by urinary tract infection should be investigated with a renal/bladder sonogram and a voiding cystourethrogram (to detect structural problems (Galejs & Kass 1999).

Treatment

- Oral antibiotics (commenced prior to bacterial culture results)
- Antibiotics specific to culture and sensitivity
- Nonsteroidal anti-inflammatory drugs (NSAIDs).

Pain and swelling generally resolve within a week.

At interview

The man should be informed of the need for urgent treatment. There is also a need for him to inform his sexual partner(s) should laboratory tests attribute the source of infection to a sexually transmitted organism.

ORCHITIS

Orchitis is an acute inflammatory condition of the testis usually associated with infection elsewhere in the body (e.g. pneumonia, scarlet fever, tuberculosis and syphilis) or scrotal trauma. Untreated male carriers of *Chlamydia trachomatis* (the commonest curable sexually transmitted pathogen in the UK) may present with complications of the infection, e.g. epidydimo-orchitis (Thompson et al 2001).

Orchitis is also a complication of mumps (infectious parotitis), occurring in approximately 18% of men. The mumps virus is excreted in urine. The infection may be unilateral or bilateral.

Since the introduction of a vaccine against the mumps virus there is a diminished risk for mumps and its complications. However, in cases of scrotal swelling mumps orchitis should still be considered.

Presentation (orchitis)

- Severe testicular pain
- Testicular swelling
- Tender to touch
- Red scrotum
- Chills and fever.

Complications

- Hydrocele
- Abscess
- Although spermatogenesis is irrevocably damaged in approximately 30% of cases the testes continue to have adequate hormonal function.

Treatment

- Bed rest
- Scrotal support
- Local cooling
- Systemic treatment with non-steroidal anti-inflammatory drugs
- Analgesia.

Bacterial infection

For bacterial orchitis ciprofloxacin or clavulanic acid/amoxicillin has been prescribed as appropriate.

VARICOCELE

Incompetent valves within testicular veins cause the vessels to dilate along the tract of the spermatic cord, resulting in varicoceles. The condition does not occur before puberty because testicular blood flow in prepubescent boys remains relatively low. A combination of incompetent valves and increased testicular blood flow after puberty results in veins becoming clinically apparent in adolescence. Varicocele is present in approximately 15% of men. The incidence is highest in males between 15 and 35 years. Although this condition is the most commonly diagnosed cause of male infertility, nearly two thirds of men with varicoceles remain fertile, this phenomenon remains unexplained. The pathogenesis of infertility in this condition is poorly understood. The presence of varicocele is readily diagnosed on examination.

On examination

- When palpated, varicoceles feel like a bag of worms.
- The veins distend when abdominal pressure increases (Valsalva's manoeuvre or standing).
- Veins disappear when patient is recumbent.
- The left side is more affected.
- Varicoceles are usually asymptomatic.

Investigations

- Real time ultrasound
- Spermatic venography
- Scrotopenogram.

Treatment

Most experts agree that only clinically apparent varicoceles should be treated. Along with improving fertility, surgery relieves the sensation of scrotal heaviness. Using a Cochrane review and critical analysis of research, Sandlow (2004, p. 967–968) concludes that: 'Varicoceles continue to stimulate controversy among reproductive experts. Despite conflicting evidence from both randomised and non-randomised trials, clinical experience still favours the surgical treatment of clinical varicoceles in men with infertility.' Sandlow adds: 'Although few randomised controlled trials show the benefit of treating varicocele related infertility, many non-randomised studies support this concept.'

Surgical approaches to treatment

- Open microsurgical methods (few complications)
- laparoscopic varix ligation.

N.B. Radiological ablation is often reserved for failed surgical approaches (rare).

SPERMATOCELE

Spermatocele is an accumulation of dead and liquefied sperm, often found at the head of the epididymis, in the form of a cyst. Spermatoceles occur most commonly in the fourth and fifth decades in men (Gondos & Wong 1989). The problem is entirely asymptomatic but men are often alarmed when they detect a scrotal mass on self-examination.

Spermatoceles:

- Are a benign mass
- Have unknown aetiology
- May occur after trauma or infection
- Have a poorly understood pathophysiology (possibly epididymal obstruction)
- Increase in incidence with age
- Have an incidence of 30% revealed on scrotal ultrasounds (Gondos & Wong 1989, Junnila & Lassen 1998).

Differentiation must be made between a spermatocele and other scrotal masses (e.g. tumour and varicoceles). Spermatoceles are found most often in the region of the epididymis, at the posterior of the testes. Unlike varicoceles, spermatoceles do not distend when Valsalva's manoeuvre is performed. Spermatoceles differ from epididymal cysts in that they contain sperm (if sperm is present on aspiration, then the mass is a spermatocele).

On examination

- A smooth and firm circumscribed mass is apparent, superior and posterior of the testes.
- A mass is often felt at the head of the epididymis.
- The mass is usually < 1 cm in diameter.
- These circular masses transilluminate well.

Treatment

- Surgical removal is advised if they become large and cause discomfort.
- Anticoagulants (aspirin, NSAIDs) pre- and postoperatively are contraindicated because of the risk of haemorrhage.
- Aspiration is contraindicated because leakage of sperm into scrotal tissue will cause:

—tissue irritation
—infection
—re-accumulation of sperm
* Injection of the cyst with a sclerosant agent has 30–100% success. Sclerotherapy is not performed on young men because of risk of chemical epididymitis and possible infertility.

CRYPTORCHIDISM

Incomplete or maldescent of the testes (from abdomen to scrotum in the second trimester of pregnancy) results in cryptorchidism (unilateral or bilateral). Approximately 1 in 20 boys have this problem. The John Radcliffe Hospital Cryptorchidism Study Group (1986) found cryptorchidism in 6.7% of boys at birth and 1.5% of boys at 3 months of age. The cause is poorly understood. If spontaneous descent of the testes has not occurred by 6 months of age, surgical repositioning is required (orchidopexy). Most children have the operation between 6 months and 2 years of age. If left untreated, testicular atrophy and a decrease in spermatogenesis ensue.

Cryptorchidism and testicular cancer

Data for Chilvers and Pike's (1989) study showed that 1 boy in 120 with an undescended testis developed a testicular malignancy. The study by Forman et al (1994) confirmed previous reports correlating cryptorchidism and cancer. Performing orchidopexy at younger ages is thought to reduce the risk of testicular cancer.

INGUINAL HERNIA

Inguinal hernias are the most common type of hernias and they are far more common in males than in females. In men the herniation occurs at the point of weakness in the abdominal wall where the spermatic cord emerges. A hernia will not heal itself and men postponing consultation with medical or nursing staff run the risk of having part of their bowel included in the herniation (strangulated hernia). Fitzgibbons et al (2003) concluded that watchful waiting might be an option for management of inguinal hernia but a trial of compared outcomes was needed. Surgical treatment is the preferred option (herniorrhaphy). The weakened tissue is reinforced (hernioplasty) with surgical wire, fascia or mesh.

Examination

- Inspect the inguinal and femoral areas for protrusions.
- Inspect these areas when the patient is recumbent and standing.
- When the patient stands ask him to bear down and observe for protrusions.

Palpate the inguinal canal (using the right hand for the right side of the patient) as follows:

- Using the index finger (gloved) apply pressure to the lower portion of the scrotal sack until invagination occurs.
- Follow the spermatic cord up into the inguinal ring.
- Ask the patient to strain or cough.
- Note if herniating mass descends to finger tip (Bates et al 1995).

Surgical approaches

Nearly a decade ago debate over the cost effectiveness of laparoscopic hernia repair rested on the need for larger clinical trials before the technique was to be widely adopted (Lawrence et al 1995). Bloor et al (2003) note that although there is now strong evidence of the benefits to be gained from laparoscopic procedures, there is a lack of uptake by surgeons. Kingsnorth (2004) enters the debate by pointing out:

> Laparoscopic surgery has not affected surgery for inguinal hernia appreciably because of the increased costs and the reluctance of general surgeons to learn this complex procedure to correct a minor abnormality. Improvements in the delivery and quality of inguinal hernia surgery in the future will depend on the development of improved prosthetic mesh materials to reduce the incidence of chronic groin pain, which is now higher than recurrence rates.

Postoperative advice following open hernia repair

- Don't perform activities that cause discomfort.
- Ambulate early to prevent complications.
- Avoid driving for some days depending on vehicle type (check insurance validity post surgery).
- Office type employees can return to work after 2–3 weeks.
- Most heavy manual workers can return to work after 3–4 weeks. Return to lighter duties at first.

BALANITIS

Balanitis is an acute or chronic inflammation of the penis glans and prepuce (foreskin). Balanitis is caused by poor hygiene where bacteria and cellular debris (smegma) and secretions are allowed to collect under the prepuce. These conditions usually occur in men with phimosis or a large redundant prepuce.

On examination

- Erythema
- Exudate
- Ulceration of prepuce in chronic form.

Treatment

- Bacterial cultures and antibiotics based on sensitivity

BALANITIS XEROTICA OBLITERANS

Balanitis xerotica obliterans (BXO) is a chronic inflammatory process resulting in sclerotic epithelial changes of the glans penis, prepuce and urethral meatus individually or collectively. Early diagnosis and treatment of BXO are very important in preventing the urological complications of the diseases such as urethral stricture.

In children, stenosis of the urethral meatus requires meatal dilatation, meatotomy followed by regular dilatation. Where inflammation is advanced and the stricture severe, a meatoplasty is performed. Searles and MacKinnon (2004) have demonstrated the effectiveness of regular dilation of the urethral meatus being taught successfully to boys or their families at home, thus avoiding repeated hospital attendance and often general anaesthesia.

Most of the cases of BXO are seen in the third to fifth decades of life. Das and Tunuguntla (2000) advise that meatal stenosis, phimosis, scar adhesions, fissures, erosions of glans and prepuce and involvement of the urethra are indications for surgical treatment.

Surgery

Surgery appears to be the only method of treatment for relieving the symptoms of advanced disease. Modified circumcision, with total removal of inner preputial layer, definitively relieves phimosis without any recurrence (Das & Tunuguntla 2000).

Laser treatment

Hrebinko (1996) reports that circumferential carbon dioxide laser vaporisation monotherapy shows promise in treatment of meatal stenosis associated with balanitis xerotica obliterans.

Topical steroids

Applying a potent topical steroid affects improvement in balanitis xerotica obliterans in the histologically early and intermediate stages of disease, and may inhibit further worsening in the late stage (Kiss et al 2001).

PHIMOSIS

Phimosis is a tightness in the prepuce (foreskin) preventing its retraction over the penile glans. The incidence of phimosis is difficult to state, as there are various interpretations of the definition related to when retraction of the foreskin should occur naturally with age and whether or not a pathological process is in action. Sometimes the retracted foreskin is unable to be returned because of tightness, this is called paraphimosis. Acute paraphimosis causes swelling and pain and is a urologic emergency requiring reduction of the foreskin through surgical or nonsurgical methods. The risk of phimosis as an indication for prophylactic circumcision has been the topic of debate since the late 1940s (Gairdner 1949).

At interview

The patient may complain of :
● Pain with erection or during intercourse
● Difficulty in getting his foreskin to retract
● Difficulty in returning foreskin after retraction.

Circumcision

Paraphimosis is one of the most common reasons for adult circumcision (Holman & Stuessi 1999). Dewan's (2003) review of the data from England and Australia indicated that whilst phimosis is the most frequently given reason for circumcision in young boys much of this surgery might be unnecessary. Spilsbury et al (2003) concluded that the rate of circumcision to treat phimosis in Western Australian boys, aged less than 15 years, was seven times the expected incidence rate for phimosis. Many boys are circumcised before reaching 5 years of age, despite phimosis being rare in this age group.

Steroid treatment

The efficacy of topical steroid (beta methasone) was trialed by Wright (1994) with the result that satisfactory retractability of the foreskin, appropriate for the boys' age, was achieved in 80% of patients (n = 111). In 10%, circumcision was performed because of failure of treatment and a further 10% refused circumcision. Successful treatment depended upon the presence of a normal, supple foreskin at the outset of the study, and on parental adherence to treatment.

CANCER OF THE PENIS

Cancer of the penis is a rare disease in Western countries and almost completely limited to men who are not circumcised in childhood. The prevention of this form of cancer by circumcision has been a central factor supporting arguments for male infant circumcision. However, there was a steady fall between 1940 and 1990 in cancer of the penis in Denmark, where the population of males is virtually uncircumcised (cumulative national circumcision rate of around 1.6% by the age of 15 years). Frisch et al's (1995) study showed a declining incidence of penis cancer in Denmark, despite consistently low rates of circumcision. This suggests that other factors may reduce the risk of cancer of the penis. However, uncircumcised males with foreskins affected by other conditions may be at higher risk. Phimosis was observed in 75% of men with squamous cell carcinoma (SCC) of the penis and it is the most common structural abnormality associated with this tumour (Grossman 1992).

Cause

Although syphilis was thought to be causative in the aetiology of penile cancer, this has been rejected and superseded by evidence that the human papillomavirus (HPV 16 and to a lesser extent HPV 18) triggers the cancer (Strohmeyer 1993, Cupp et al 1995, Frisch et al 1996). Squamous cell carcinoma is the most common tumour of the penis and the cancer commonly appears in patients after the sixth decade. Prognosis is poor when nodal metastases appear.

At interview

- Patients may report a non tender nodule.
- Any persistent penile sores should be considered suspicious.

On examination

- Indurated nodule or ulcer
- Non tender

Treatment

Therapy of penis cancer is a balance between organ preservation and radical surgery. Soria et al (1997) report on a large series of patients with squamous cell carcinoma of the penis, describing prognostic factors, survival and therapeutic results.

The following conclusions about treatment methods have been extrapolated from Soria et al (1997):

- Radical surgery (penile amputation) gives the best control of the primary tumour, but it is mutilating.
- Conservative therapies (laser, radiotherapy, and particularly brachytherapy) are an attractive option.
- Management of lymph nodes is essential for improving survival even when conservative therapy is used to treat the primary tumour.
- Management of only regional lymph nodes is extremely controversial.
- More than half of patients are responsive to modern poly-chemotherapy combinations. However, the benefits are transient and chemotherapy alone is not curative for metastatic disease.

PEYRONIE'S DISEASE

Peyronie's disease is an uncommon condition primarily affecting men between 45 and 60 years of age, although an age range of 18–80 years has been reported (Fitkin & Ho 1999). This is a localised connective tissue disorder characterised by the formation of fibrous lumps (scarring) within the erectile tissue of the penis (tunica albuginea). The scar feels like a ridge and is usually located on the dorsal midline of the shaft of the penis. Scarring causes tissue contraction and subsequent accentuation of the normal curve of the penis and possibly painful erections (mostly in the initial phase of the disease).

Cause

Although trauma to the erect penis is thought to be causal, there is no clear cause.

Clinical features

Men normally seek medical advice because of:

- Penile lumps
- Curvature of the shaft of the penis on erection
- Painful erection
- Unsatisfactory penetration of the vagina (soft erections).

Implications for practice

Reassure the patient that:

- The symptoms are not associated with an STI.
- The lumps are unlikely to indicate cancer.
- In many cases the problem resolves without treatment.
- Inform the patient of treatments for softening of the scar using:
  — vitamin E cream
  — ultrasound
  — corticosteroid injections.

Surgical treatment

If severe, the curvature of the penis can be rectified by surgery that shortens the side of the penis opposite from the scar tissue. Alternatively, the scar tissue is replaced by grafting healthy tissue to the affected area.

In severe cases a prosthesis is implanted to help straighten the penis and help make it firm enough for sexual intercourse to occur. Occasionally surgery can result in scarring, making the condition worse.

References

Bates B, Bickley LS, Hoekelman RA 1995 A guide to physical examination, 6th edn., Lippincott

Bloor K, Freemantle N, Khadjesari Z et al 2003 Impact of NICE guidance on laparoscopic surgery for inguinal hernias: analysis of interrupted time series. British Medical Journal 326(7389): 578

Chilvers C, Pike MC 1989 Epidemiology of undescended testis. In: Oliver RTD, Blandy JP, Hope-Stone HF (eds) Urological and genital cancer. Blackwell, Oxford, p 306–321

Cupp MR, Malek RS, Goellner JR et al 1995 The detection of human papillomavirus deoxyribonucleic acid in intraepithelial, in situ, verrucous and invasive carcinoma of the penis. Journal of Urology 154(3): 1024–1029

Das S, Tunuguntla HS 2000 Balanitis xerotica obliterans – a review. World Journal of Urology 18(6): 382–387

Davenport M 1996a ABC of general paediatric surgery: inguinal hernia, hydrocele, and the undescended testis. British Medical Journal 312(7030): 564–567

Davenport M 1996b ABC of general surgery in children: acute problems of the scrotum. British Medical Journal 312(7028): 435–437

Dewan PA 2003 Treating phimosis. Medical Journal of Australia 178(4): 148–150

Fitkin J, Ho GT 1999 Peyronie's disease: current management. American Family Physician 60(2): 549–552, 554

Fitzigibbons RJ, Jonasson O, Gibbs J et al 2003 The development of a clinical trial to determine if watchful waiting is an acceptable alternative to routine herniorrhaphy for patients with minimal or no hernia symptoms. Journal of the American College of Surgeons 196(5): 737–742

Forman D, Pike MC, Davey G et al 1994 Aetiology of testicular cancer: association with congenital abnormalities, age at puberty, infertility, and exercise. British Medical Journal 308(6941): 1393–1399

Frisch M, Friss S, Kjaer S et al 1995 Falling incidence of penis cancer in an uncircumcised population (Denmark 1943–1990). British Medical Journal 311(7018): 1471

Frisch M, Jorgensen BB, Friis S et al 1996 Syphilis and the risk of penis cancer. Sexually Transmitted Diseases 23(6): 471–474

Gairdner D 1949 The fate of the foreskin. British Medical Journal 2: 1433–1437

Galejs LE, Kass EJ 1999 Diagnosis and treatment of the acute scrotum. American Family Physician. Article 817. American Academy of Family Physicians. Online. Available: http://www.aafp.org/afp/990215ap/817.html.

Gondos B, Wong TW 1989 Non-neoplastic diseases of the testis and epididymis. In: Murphy WM (ed) Urological pathology. WB Saunders, Philadelphia, p 249–313

Grossman HB 1992 Premalignant and early carcinomas of the penis and scrotum. Urological Clinics of North America 19(2): 221–225

Holman JR, Stuessi KA 1999 Adult circumcision. American Family Physician. American Academy of Family Physicians. Online. Available: http://www.aafp.org/afp/990315ap/1514.html

Hrebinko RL 1996 Circumferential laser vaporization for severe meatal stenosis secondary to balanitis xerotica obliterans. Journal of Urology 156(5): 1735–1736

John Radcliffe Hospital Cryptorchidism Study Group 1986 Cryptorchidism: an apparent substantial increase since 1960. British Medical Journal 293(6559): 1401–1404

Junnila J, Lassen P 1998 Testicular masses. American Family Physicians 57(4). American Academy of Family Physicians. Online. Available: http://www.aafp.org/afp/980215ap/junnila.htm

Kingsnorth A 2004 Treating inguinal hernias. British Medical Journal 328(7431): 59–60

Kiss A, Csontai A, Pirot L et al 2001 The response of balanitis xerotica obliterans to local steroid application compared with placebo in children. Journal of Urology 165(1): 219–220

Lawrence K, McWhinnie D, Goodwin A et al 1995 Randomised controlled trial of laparoscopic versus open repair of inguinal hernia: early results. British Medical Journal 311(7011): 981–985

Luscombe CJ, Coppinger SMV, Mountford PJ et al 1996 Diagnosing testicular torsion. British Medical Journal 312(7042): 1358–1359

Pentyala S, Lee J, Yalamanchili P et al 2001 Testicular torsion: a review. Journal of Lower Genital Tract Disease 31(1): 38–47

Sandlow J 2004 Pathogenesis and treatment of varicoceles. British Medical Journal 328(7746): 967–968

Searles JM, MacKinnon AE 2004 Home-dilatation of the urethral meatus in boys. British Journal of Urology International 93(4): 596–597

Soria JC, Fizazi K, Piron D et al 1997 Squamous cell carcinoma of the penis: multivariate analysis of prognostic factors and natural history in monocentric study with a conservative policy. Annals of Oncology 8(11): 1089–1098

Spilsbury K, Semmens JB, Wisniewski ZS et al 2003 Routine circumcision for phimosis and other medical indications in Western Australian boys. Medical Journal of Australia 178(4): 155–158

Strohmeyer T 1993 Penis cancer. The etiological importance of papilloma viruses. Hautarzt 44(3): 133–134

Thompson C, Macdonald M, Sutherland S 2001 A family cluster of *Chlamydia trachomatis* infection. British Medical Journal 322(7300): 1473–1474

Wright JE 1994 The treatment of childhood phimosis with topical steroid. Australian and New Zealand Journal of Surgery 64(5): 327–328

Further reading

Homayoon K, Suhre CD, Steinhardt GF 2004 Epididymal cysts in children: natural history. Journal of Urology 171(3): 1274–1276

Junnila J, Lassen P 1998 Testicular masses. American Family Physician 7: 215

Mycyk M, Moyer P 2001 Orchitis. Emedecine. Online. Available: http://www.emedicine.com/emerg/topic 344.htm

Sugita Y, Clarnette TD, Cooke-Yarborough C et al 1999 Testicular and paratesticular tumours in children: 30 years' experience. Australian and New Zealand Journal of Surgery 69(7): 505–508

Resources

Ehrlich R, Alter G 1998 Reconstructive and plastic surgery of the external genitalia: adult and pediatric. Saunders Philadelphia *Ehrlich and Alter have produced the first book in over 20 years addressing both urologic and plastic surgery aspects of genital reconstruction in a single volume. Its in-depth, state-of-the-art coverage includes an introduction to plastic surgery principles and external genitalia anatomy, vaginal reconstruction, male to female gender reassignment, total phalloplasty, aesthetic genital surgery, Peyronie's disease, and more.*

Index

Page numbers in *italics* refer to figures and tables.